Fractures of the
facial skeleton

Fractures of the facial skeleton

Michael Perry

Consultant Maxillofacial Surgeon, London North West Healthcare Regional Maxillofacial Unit and Regional Trauma Centre (Northwick Park Hospital, Harrow and St Mary's Hospital, London, UK)

Andrew Brown

Honorary Consultant Maxillofacial Surgeon, Regional Maxillofacial Unit, Queen Victoria Hospital, East Grinstead, UK

Peter Banks

Honorary Consultant Maxillofacial Surgeon, Regional Maxillofacial Unit, Queen Victoria Hospital, East Grinstead, UK

SECOND EDITION

WILEY Blackwell

Library of Congress Cataloging-in-Publication Data

Perry, Michael (Surgeon) author.
   Fractures of the facial skeleton / Michael Perry, Andrew Brown, Peter Banks. – 2nd edition.
      p. ; cm.
   Preceded by: Fractures of the facial skeleton / Peter Banks and Andrew Brown. 2001.
   Includes bibliographical references and index.
   ISBN 978-1-119-96766-8 (pbk. : alk. paper)
   I. Brown, Andrew (Andrew K.), author. II. Banks, Peter, 1936- , author. III. Banks, Peter, 1936- .
Fractures of the facial skeleton. Preceded by (work): IV. Title.
   [DNLM: 1.   Facial Bones–injuries. 2.   Skull Fractures. 3.   Facial Injuries–therapy. 4.   Fracture
Fixation.   WE 706]
   RD523
   617.5′2044–dc23

                                                                    2015006389

A catalogue record for this book is available from the British Library.

Cover credit: Image courtesy of Michael Perry

Wiley also publishes its books in a variety of electronic formats. Some content that appears in print may not be available in electronic books.

Typeset in 8.5/12pt MeridienLTStd by Laserwords Private Limited, Chennai, India

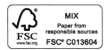

Contents

Preface

It is now more than a decade since the first edition of this book was published and its popularity has justified several reprints. The original concept was to have a small book that was not simply an exam orientated text for postgraduate students in maxillofacial surgery. That concept bears repetition: to summarize what is accepted and well known while providing detailed debate in areas where controversy remains. The then authors hoped it would appeal to all surgical specialties involved in facial trauma to further accurate diagnosis and an understanding of the principles of management. This new edition has expanded the section on general trauma management and the place of maxillofacial injuries within that spectrum. To that end there is now a third author with wide experience in this field.

The development and improvement in maxillofacial trauma management in recent years is hugely related to advances in imaging. Surgical techniques, however, have not undergone equivalent dramatic change and in some cases promising ideas and materials have not proved as useful as expected. On the credit side, however, the overall functional and cosmetic outcome for injuries that involve the dentition has advanced as a result of implant technology.

This edition still contains brief descriptions of a few techniques that may only be regularly employed in those parts of the world where easy access to plating equipment continues to be limited. Nevertheless, there are some methods previously in common use which are now clearly obsolete; any mention of them in this revised text is solely to show their limitations or where an historical comparison appeared useful.

Although this book is first and foremost about the management of fractures of the facial skeleton and the dentition, the subject is impossible to divorce from associated soft tissue injury and these sections have been expanded without attempting to be comprehensive.

Acknowledgements

A number of figures are taken from *Atlas of Operative Maxillofacial Trauma Surgery*. Michael Perry and Simon Holmes (Eds): Springer; 2014, and reproduced with kind permission.

Figures 7.10 a–e have been kindly provided by Kenneth Sneddon, Consultant Maxillofacial Surgeon, Queen Victoria Hospital, East Grinstead and illustrate a case operated on by him.

Figure 7.18 has been kindly provided by Jeremy Collyer, Consultant Maxillofacial Surgeon, Queen Victoria Hospital, East Grinstead and are pre-operative images of a patient under his care.

Figures 8.4. 8.5, 8.6 and 8.8 have been kindly provided by Malcolm Cameron, Consultant Maxillofacial Surgeon, Addenbrooke's Hospital, Cambridge.

CHAPTER 1

Facial trauma: incidence, aetiology and principles of treatment

Facial trauma is a challenging area of clinical practice. By its very nature, the highly visible effects it can have on both the function and aesthetics of the face means that any repair that is less than perfect will be all too apparent. Injuries to the nasoethmoid region are especially noticeable – the medial canthus needs only to drift a millimetre or so to become obvious. However, fractures are just one component of the spectrum of 'maxillofacial injuries'. They are variably associated with injuries to the overlying soft tissues and neighbouring structures such as the eyes, lacrimal apparatus, nasal airways, paranasal sinuses, tongue and various sensory and motor nerves.

The bones and tissues of the face support and maintain a number of key functions, including those relating to the oral cavity, nasal cavity and orbits. Not surprisingly, injuries to the face can have a major cosmetic impact and even so-called 'minor' injuries if poorly treated can result in significant disability and an unsightly appearance. When fractures extend into the skull base and involve the intracranial contents they are usually referred to as 'craniofacial' injuries. These will often require combined management with a neurosurgeon. Facial trauma can vary in severity therefore from a simple crack in a bone to major disruption of the entire facial skeleton with associated severe soft tissue injury.

Most facial injuries occur following relatively low energy impacts and require relatively straightforward treatment. However, despite high patient satisfaction rates, less than perfect results are still common. Clinicians treating these injuries should strive for the ideal goal of returning the patient to their pre-injury form and function. Unfortunately in many cases, especially when high energy injuries have resulted in both comminution of the facial skeleton and significant soft tissue damage, this cannot always be achieved. Despite major developments in the fields of tissue healing,

biomaterials and surgical technology, there is still room for improvement.

Although fractures of the facial skeleton are common, they can easily be overlooked when accompanied by soft tissue swelling or lacerations. Delay in diagnosis can contribute to the likelihood of residual deformity and all doctors working in emergency departments should therefore be able to recognize these injuries, understand their significance and be familiar with basic management. Fractures of the lower jaw or alveolus may also present to a dental surgeon in general practice, or very rarely be a complication of a difficult tooth extraction. An understanding of facial fractures, as well as other facial injuries, has a practical application for many specialists therefore, and is not just of relevance to those studying for higher qualifications or those pursuing a career in specialist surgery.

When considering the topic of facial fractures parallels can be drawn with orthopaedic surgery. In a sense, management of facial trauma can be regarded as 'facial orthopaedics' and as such requires the same core knowledge of fracture management and application of similar treatment principles. These include an understanding of fracture healing, principles of fixation and an appreciation of the importance of the 'soft tissue envelope'. However, facial surgeons will also need to draw on their specialist aesthetic skills to ensure the best possible results, facilitating this by being as anatomically precise as possible.

Incidence

When considering trauma in all its forms maxillofacial injuries are not particularly common, although it is difficult to arrive at any accurate estimate of their global

Fractures of the Facial Skeleton, Second Edition. Michael Perry, Andrew Brown and Peter Banks.
© 2015 John Wiley & Sons, Ltd. Published 2015 by John Wiley & Sons, Ltd.

incidence. Estimates vary considerably both within and between countries. Reported incidences may also be skewed, depending on local referral pathways. Nasal fractures, for instance, are commonly treated by plastic surgeons and otorhinolaryngologists as well as oral and maxillofacial surgeons. As a result they may not be fully captured by any single database. There will also be a variation in the number of fractures treated by any particular specialist unit depending on geographical location, the demographics of the catchment population and seasonal factors. Generally speaking, the most common facial fractures are nasal and mandibular fractures, followed by injuries to the zygoma, maxilla and orbit. Dentoalveolar fractures are also common but may not present to specialist centres, so accurate figures are not widely available. Finally, the terminology used for recording injuries may add to the confusion about fracture incidence. For example, the term 'middle third fracture' is not anatomically precise and may be used to include fractures of the midface, orbito-zygomatic complex and fractures of the nose.

In one large study of patients sustaining injuries as a result of personal assault approximately 80% of all fractures and 66% of all lacerations were facial. Other prospective studies of severely injured patients have shown that a significant number of maxillofacial injuries may also be associated with life-threatening injuries elsewhere. Of these patients, approximately one fifth subsequently died while in hospital. This frequency of coexisting injuries may have major implications when considering transfer to specialist centres.

Aetiology

In many countries the common causes of fractures of the facial bones are interpersonal violence, sporting injuries, falls, motor vehicle collisions (road traffic accidents) and industrial or agricultural trauma. For the first 30 years after the World War II, motor vehicle collisions (MVC) were the major cause of maxillofacial injuries, accounting for between 35 and 60% of fractures of the facial bones. Following the introduction of alcohol, seat belt and crash helmet legislation, these patterns dramatically changed. Many longitudinal studies from countries such as the Netherlands, Germany and the UK have reported that economically prosperous countries have shown a striking reduction in motor vehicle collisions as a specific

cause of facial injuries, while at the same time there has been an increase in interpersonal violence and sports related injuries.

The incidences and causes of facial bone fractures are mostly influenced by:
1 Geography.
2 Social trends.
3 Alcohol and drug abuse.
4 Road traffic legislation.
5 Seasons.

Geography
Numerous studies have now shown clear relationships between urban living and facial injuries, possibly linked to alcohol consumption and social deprivation. Not surprisingly agricultural-type injuries are more commonly seen in rural communities. In developing countries where there is a rapid increase in road traffic, motor vehicle related trauma is still a major cause of fractures. In some countries, notably in some states in the USA, gunshot trauma now exceeds road traffic accidents as a cause of facial injuries.

Social trends
In more recent years in urban areas, interpersonal violence has accounted for an increasing proportion of facial bone fractures. This includes domestic abuse. Data from a number of centres around the world suggests that interpersonal violence now accounts for more than half of all facial injuries seen in emergency departments. In the United Kingdom between 1977 and 1987 there was a 47% increase in maxillofacial injuries caused by assault, while simultaneously there was a 34% decrease in road accident victims with facial bone fractures. The relative incidence of other facial injuries, such as lacerations, has also been influenced by these trends.

Alcohol and drug abuse
In many countries alcohol and drug abuse are now major factors in the aetiology of traumatic injuries. Maxillofacial injuries are commoner in young men than any other group and to a large extent this is a reflection of the increased alcohol consumption by this section of society and the violence that may ensue. Indeed it has been said that 'the combination of alcohol and testosterone is a potent mix'. Alcohol and drugs may also be a significant factor in maxillofacial injuries sustained

by road users. The influence of alcohol on maxillofacial trauma was clearly demonstrated in a large prospective study of 6114 facial injuries presenting over a period of one week to 163 UK emergency departments. Of these, 40% of facial injuries were caused by falls, a large proportion of which were in children under five years and occurred within the home. However, 24% of the injuries were caused by interpersonal violence, mainly in young adults. In this group alcohol consumption was implicated in some way in 55%. Only 5% of facial injuries were caused by road traffic accidents (RTA) with 15% of victims having consumed alcohol. The 15–25 age group suffered the greatest number of facial injuries due to either assault or RTA and had the highest number of injuries associated with alcohol consumption. Overall at least 22% of all facial injuries in all age groups were related to alcohol consumption within 4 hours of the injury.

Road traffic legislation

Vehicle safety design has been influenced both by research and legislation, and in many countries the use of seat belt restraint has now been made compulsory in law. Seat belts have resulted in a dramatic decrease in injuries overall and severe injury in particular and that general trend has been reflected in the incidence of facial injury. The beneficial effects of improved car design and the use of seat belts are now well accepted, although there is some evidence that seat belts are not entirely effective in reducing the incidence of mandibular fractures. Air bags have also been associated with particular injury patterns to the orbit and globe. Interestingly, enforced low speed limits do not appear to carry the same benefit for facial fractures compared with other types of injury. Presumably, as a result of these changes, many patients who would have otherwise died are now surviving. Helmets are also mandatory for cyclists and motorcyclists alike in many countries, although most cycle helmets are primarily designed for brain protection and offer little effective protection to the face.

Seasons

Facial fractures show a seasonal variation in most temperate zones, which reflects the increased traffic and increased urban violence during summer months and the adverse road conditions in the presence of snow and ice in mid-winter. Sporting injuries also show a marked seasonal variation. Seasonal affective disorders and failed attempts at suicide may make a very small contribution in some countries.

Principles of treatment

Surgical anatomy
The facial skeleton

Understanding the applied surgical anatomy of the facial skeleton and its associated structures is extremely important in the assessment and management of facial fractures. Specific fracture patterns are well known to commonly occur and the effects of displaced bone fragments, notably at the skull base and orbital apex, can dramatically affect risks and outcomes. Traditionally the facial skeleton has been divided into an upper, middle and lower third. The lower third is the mandible. The upper third is formed by the frontal bone. The middle third is the region extending downwards from the frontal bone to the level of the upper teeth, or if the patient is edentulous the upper alveolus. However, this arbitrary division now has much less role to play in modern management. The terminology used can also sometimes be a little confusing. Fractures of the middle third of the face are often referred to as 'upper jaw fractures' or 'fractures of the maxilla'. However, in view of the fact that the adjacent bones are almost invariably involved, these terms are not strictly accurate. It is perhaps better to use the terms 'midfacial' and 'fractures of the midface' (Fig. 1.1).

From a functional point of view, an interesting and teleological question is, 'Why do some animals have sinuses?' A number of theories exist, but the answer is still unclear. One suggestion is that the skeleton of the midface has evolved into a protective 'crumple zone', functioning much like the chassis of a modern car. As such it acts as a cushion, absorbing the energy of any cranially directed impacts coming from an anterior or anterolateral direction. The midface can be considered as a fragile 'matchbox' sitting below and in front of a hard shell containing the brain. In this respect it differs markedly from the rigid projection of the mandible below (Fig. 1.2). The midfacial bones have the capacity to absorb impact energy, thereby protecting the brain and conferring a survival advantage. Any impact directly applied to the cranium may be sufficient to cause severe brain injury. However, the same force applied to the

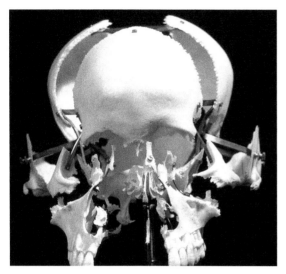

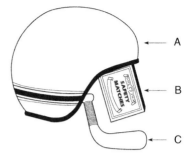

Figure 1.2 Diagrammatic representation of the relative strength of the skull and facial bones. The 'matchbox' like structure of the midface cushions the force of impact (B), whereas a blow to the skull is transmitted directly to the intracranial contents (A). An impact to the mandible (C) is transmitted indirectly to the cranial base. Damage to the brain may be prevented by protective fracture of the condylar neck, which is represented here as the handle of a bent baseball bat.

Figure 1.1 Anatomical specimen showing the bones of the mid and upper face separated and mounted to show their complex inter-relationship. Note that the bones of the midfacial skeleton are all relatively fragile. From above downwards they are the perpendicular plate of the ethmoid, with paired lacrimal bones, nasal bones, palatine bones, maxillae and inferior conchae. The zygomatic bones are shown laterally. The midline vomer is missing. (Courtesy of the Wellcome Museum of Anatomy and Pathology, Royal College of Surgeons of England.)

midface is cushioned as the bones collapse. In many cases the force is absorbed to such an extent that it may not even lead to loss of consciousness. Of course the price of surviving such an impact may be considerable damage to the bones and soft tissues of the face. In those cases where the mandible absorbs the entire impact the cushioning effect is reduced and brain injury can result, as with a boxer's knockout punch. However, occasionally one or both condyles fracture following a blow to the chin. This mechanism may afford some degree of protection to the brain stem and upper cervical cord passing through the rigid foramen magnum.

The midface is therefore so ordered that it can simultaneously withstand the forces of mastication and at the same time provide protection for vital structures, notably the brain and eye. This design has evolved as a result of Wolff's law, which states that healthy bone will remodel in response to the functional loads to which it is subjected. In the face most of this loading is related to biting and chewing forces. Where bone is not needed, it is resorbed. Thus, the midface contains the minimal amount of bone required to provide support

and protection of several important organs, including the eyes and upper respiratory/olfactory tract.

The bones of the midface can therefore be thought of as a series of vertical and horizontal bony struts or 'buttresses' surrounding the sinuses, eyes and uppermost part of the respiratory tract. Joining these buttresses together is wafer-thin bone. The forces of mastication are thus distributed round the nasal airway, globes and paranasal sinuses as they pass upwards to the relatively rigid skull base (Fig. 1.3). Experiments have supported this theory. Fractures of the midface have been shown to occur with forces between one-fifth and one-third of those required to produce simple fractures of the mandible. Although this 'crumple zone' type arrangement may appear to have an obvious survival advantage collapse of the buttresses can result in significant displacement of the tissues. The midfacial bones as a whole have a very low tolerance to impact forces. The nasal bones are least resistant, followed by the zygomatic arch, while the maxilla itself is very sensitive to horizontal impacts.

The upper third of the facial skeleton is chiefly the frontal bone, which forms the superior orbital margin and orbital roof. From here, the base of the skull extends backwards and downwards at approximately 45° from the frontal bone. The midfacial complex articulates with this slope and is effectively suspended from the skull base. In the midline the cribriform plate of the ethmoid makes contact with the meninges of the brain and transmits the olfactory nerves (Fig. 1.4). High energy impacts

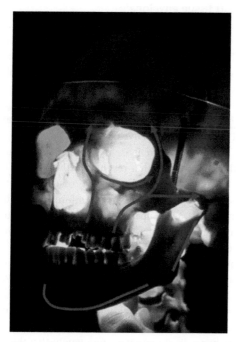

Figure 1.3 Transilluminated skull and facial bones demonstrating the thick buttresses of bone that distribute the forces of mastication within the skeleton of the midface. The much stronger bone of the mandible is also clearly evident. (Reproduced with kind permission of Springer Science+Business Media.)

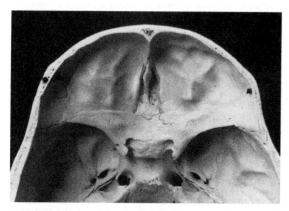

Figure 1.4 View of the anterior cranial base showing the cribriform plate of the ethmoid with the olfactory nerve foramina and midline crista galli. This fragile bone is fractured in high midface Le Fort type and severe naso-orbito-ethmoid injuries. Damage to the underlying dura may result in cerebrospinal fluid rhinorrhoea.

can result in the middle third of the face being sheared off the cranial base with displacement downwards and backwards along this plane. As a result, the upper posterior teeth impact on the lower ones and prop open the bite. Clinically, this results in an elongated face and an anterior open bite (see Fig. 3.12 in Chapter 3). In severe cases there may be significant swelling and severe bleeding. Airway compromise may occur, particularly in the supine patient.

In most fractures of the facial skeleton the frontal and sphenoid bones, including the greater and lesser wings, are not usually fractured. In fact, they are protected to a considerable extent by the cushioning effect achieved by the midface already mentioned. Fractures of the cranial components tend to occur following direct blows to these bones.

The protective buttresses also define the three dimensional shape of the face. When it comes to planning the treatment of the injured facial skeleton attention to the buttresses is important. Anatomical reduction is essential if precise three-dimensional re-establishment of facial height, width and projection is to be achieved (Fig. 1.5). Attention to the nasal septum is also an important part of this and is often overlooked. Not only is the septum crucial in the development of the growing midface, but it is an important element in maintaining nasal projection and patency. A useful way to visualize the facial skeleton is to think of it like a framed picture when viewed from in front. The 'frame' is made up of the rigid frontal bone above, two vertical lateral struts made up by the lateral orbital margins and the zygomatic complex and a lower horizontal mandibular platform, which is hinged and mobile. This frame contains a complicated 'picture' made up of the multiple bones of the midface, the orbital contents, paranasal sinuses and teeth. The overlying soft tissues (the 'glass'), including the cartilaginous nasal skeleton, complete the composition. This analogy is useful. If a framed picture is damaged it is repaired in a logical order. The frame is first reconstructed followed by a detailed restoration of the contents and finally the protective glass is replaced. Although correct sequencing is important when repairing complex facial injuries, the precise order is somewhat controversial and opinions differ. One possible sequence can be represented diagrammatically using concentric circles as a guide (Fig. 1.6).

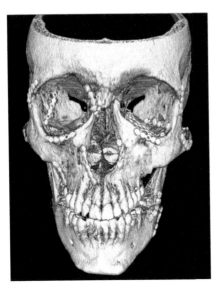

Figure 1.5 The importance of accurate anatomical reduction to restore all three dimensions of the facial skeleton. Representation of a three-dimensional CT scan of a complex facial fracture that has been reduced and treated with miniplate fixation of the main buttress areas. (Reproduced with kind permission of Springer Science+Business Media.)

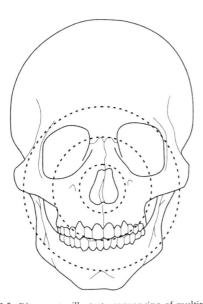

Figure 1.6 Diagram to illustrate sequencing of multiple facial fracture repair. The outer circle defines the 'frame' of stronger bones that are reduced and immobilized first (frontal bone, lateral orbital margins, zygomas and mandible). The middle circle contains the 'contents' of this 'frame' (essentially the maxillae) that are reduced and repaired next, and finally the nasal complex (inner circle) is restored.

The 'soft tissue envelope'

The healing process following a fracture can be considered under two aspects; healing of the soft tissues and healing of the bone. Correct management of the associated soft tissue injury is essential and often under-appreciated. It is not just a case of getting the bones back together. The entire healing process and subsequent rehabilitation relies heavily on the viability of the 'soft tissue envelope', more specifically its blood supply. As such it is important to be mindful that the energy force that resulted in the fracture also passed through the overlying soft tissues to get to the bone. The soft tissues are therefore injured to a varying extent, quite apart from the additional trauma of any surgical repair. Blast, crush and compound injuries are obvious examples of soft tissue injury, and lacerations do not necessarily need to be present to indicate extensive damage to the soft tissues. With most blunt trauma of course soft tissue loss and gross contamination is unusual, although the soft tissues may still be significantly damaged.

In orthopaedic surgery it is often taught that the success of fracture management depends not only on the condition of the bones and how well they are repaired, but also to a large extent on the condition of the overlying soft tissues. Consider for example two identical fractures, one of which is covered by healthy, well vascularized soft tissues, while the other is exposed through a heavily contaminated, open wound following a crush injury. Whether the fracture is in the leg, arm, mandible or midface, intuitively outcomes will be better in the first fracture than in the second. This comparison highlights the importance of the soft tissues, and in particular the blood supply, in the healing process. In this regard the mechanism of injury gives useful clues as to the likelihood of injury to the soft tissues. Take for example fractures following a single punch, being kicked by a horse, a blast injury and being shot. Each mechanism carries with it increasing amounts of kinetic energy, potentially compromising the vascularity of the tissues. The more the blood supply is compromised, the greater the chances of infection, non-healing and bone loss. Comminution in a fracture implies high energy transfer and more energy is therefore transferred to the surrounding soft tissues during the injury. Excessive movement across the fracture also has an adverse effect in healing by preventing vascularization of the bone fragments. These factors have major implications for the choice of repair.

Gunshot or missile injuries also transfer a considerable amount of energy and blast effects deep into the tissues. Ballistic injuries of this type differ from most other facial injuries. They are often heavily contaminated with extensive soft tissue disruption and tissue loss. They may also be associated with thermal injury, and the transmission of the blast effect through the tissues may result in damage at sites relatively remote from the injury. Contaminated wounds may therefore require several operations with serial debridement and packing. However, in the maxillofacial region, because of the excellent blood supply, this is only required in really heavily contaminated wounds. Management of this type of injury requires experience and judgement. If there is any doubt about tissue viability it is better to adopt a 'watch and wait policy' and delay intervention for 48 hours or so in order that non-vital tissue can declare itself.

Fracture classification

The basic orthopaedic classification of fractures as simple, open, comminuted and pathological can equally be applied to the facial skeleton.

Simple (closed)

These include fractures of the condylar process, coronoid process and ramus of the mandible, and fractures of the body of the edentulous mandible. The 'greenstick' fracture is a rare variant of the simple fracture and is found exclusively in children.

Open (compound)

Fractures of the tooth-bearing portions of the mandible and midface are nearly always open into the mouth via the periodontal membrane. More rarely, fractures may be compound through the overlying skin. Nasal and zygomatic fractures are technically 'open' into the sinonasal airway tract, but usually heal without infective complications probably due to their extensive blood supply.

Comminuted

A comminuted fracture is one where the bone is fragmented into multiple pieces. This usually requires considerably more energy than does a simple fracture. Direct violence to the mandible from penetrating sharp objects and missiles may cause limited or extensive comminution. Such fractures are usually compound and may be further complicated by bone and soft tissue loss.

Pathological

Fractures are termed pathological when they result from minimal trauma to a bone already weakened by a pre-existing pathological condition (such as osteomyelitis, neoplasms or generalized skeletal disease). In the face this is most commonly seen in the mandible.

Whilst this orthopaedic classification is applicable to the facial skeleton a more practical approach is to consider maxillofacial fractures as falling into one of two main groups:

1 Fractures without gross comminution of the bone and without significant loss of hard or soft tissue.
2 Fractures with gross comminution of the bone and with extensive loss of both hard and soft tissue.

The majority of fractures fall into the first category. Those in the second group either result from missile injuries, industrial injuries involving machinery or major road accidents, where there is direct injury from sharp objects moving at relatively high velocity. Although somewhat arbitrary, this broad division is useful because the management of the second group is entirely different from the first, both in terms of the primary assessment and repair.

Fracture healing

Fracture healing is often referred to as 'direct' or 'indirect'. These are two entirely different processes and have major implications in management. Direct healing (or primary bone healing) can only occur when there is absolute rigidity across a fracture and sufficient bone to bone contact. Growth of bone occurs across the gap and there is no callus formation. Compression across a fracture is believed to facilitate this and healing is usually rapid. Although plating techniques in orthopaedic surgery are designed to encourage direct healing, in the face this is only practically possible in the mandible. This is because direct healing requires heavy plates and large screws to achieve the necessary degree of rigidity and compression. Indirect healing is a different process and occurs across a fracture where some degree of mobility persists. This is seen in limbs treated with orthopaedic casts and is the natural healing process seen in land mammals. Initial hematoma formation is followed by the ingrowth of delicate fibrovascular tissue. Gradual ossification then occurs and the fracture is encased by 'immature bone' or callus. This is more prominent in load bearing situations and provides early stability. Once fully healed, remodelling of the callus occurs, resulting in the final trabecular or 'mature' bone. Callus formation therefore implies some degree of mobility across a fracture during healing. This type of healing is more commonly seen following repair of facial fractures, although with the newer materials fixation hardware is achieving increasingly greater degrees of rigidity.

Principles of fracture repair

In both orthopaedic surgery and maxillofacial surgery there are a number of basic principles commonly shared in fracture management. Both specialties have now moved towards open repair of most fractures, in preference to the less precise methods of closed reduction. Open repair facilitates anatomical reduction and fixation, and subsequent restoration of function. The relationship between excessive movement, poor union and infection is also well understood in both specialties. However, unlike limb fractures the repair of maxillofacial injuries can generally wait longer if necessary. This is due to the presence of the excellent blood supply to the face and, where relevant, salivary growth factors. Facial fractures can also be more extensively exposed, with less risk of infection or necrosis. Complete detachment of bone from the soft tissues (extra corporeal repair) and non-vascularized bone grafting are also possible. However, the repair of facial fractures requires a higher level of precision than most orthopaedic injuries in order to achieve optimum function and aesthetics.

Fracture fixation may be either rigid or semi-rigid. In the strictest sense rigid fixation means that there will be no movement whatsoever across the fracture site. This produces such a level of stability that direct bone healing can take place, assuming there is sufficient bone-to-bone contact. Rigid fixation therefore requires strong 'load bearing' fixation devices, usually large plates and bicortical screws. As such, these devices tend to be bulky and can only be used in the mandible. The other bones of the face are too friable to support such plates. With semi-rigid fixation there is still adequate support, although a variable amount of 'micro movement' will still occur. Much smaller so-called 'miniplates' can therefore be used.

Currently opinions differ on the amount of stability that is required for optimal healing. Rigid fixation is not as critical in the face as it is in the limbs and therefore maxillofacial fractures can be managed in several ways. Intermaxillary fixation (IMF), semi-rigid fixation and rigid fixation can all result in satisfactory healing, yet the degree of stability that each produces clearly varies.

Further reading

American College of Surgeons Committee on Trauma. *ATLS Advanced Trauma Life Support for Doctors.* 9th edn. Chicago: American College of Surgeons; 2012.

Bhrany AD. Craniomaxillofacial buttresses: anatomy and repair. *Arch Facial Plast Surg.* 2012 Nov 1;14(6):469. doi: 10.1001/arch facial.2012.906.

Giannoudis PI, Tzioupis C, Almalki T, Buckley R. Fracture healing in osteoporotic fractures: is it really different? A basic science perspective. *Injury.* 2007 Mar;38 Suppl 1:S90–99.

Kambalimath HV, Agarwal SM, Kambalimath DH, Singh M, Jain N, Michael P. Maxillofacial injuries in children: A 10 year retrospective study. *J Maxillofac Oral Surg.* 2013 Jun;12(2):140–144. doi: 10.1007/s12663–012–0402–6. Epub 2012 Aug 26.

Kraft A, Abermann E, Stigler R, Zsifkovits C, Pedross F, Kloss F, Gassner R. Craniomaxillofacial trauma: synopsis of 14,654 cases with 35,129 injuries in 15 years. *Craniomaxillofac Trauma Reconstr.* 2012 Mar;5(1):41–50.

Lee K. Global trends in maxillofacial fractures. *Craniomaxillofac Trauma Reconstr.* 2012 Dec;5(4):213–222. doi: 10.1055/s-0032–1322535. Epub 2012 Oct 18.

McAllister PI, Jenner S, Laverick S. Toxicology screening in oral and maxillofacial trauma patients. *Br J Oral Maxillofac Surg.* 2013 Dec;51(8):773–778. doi: 10.1016/j.bjoms.2013.03.017. Epub 2013 Sep 9.

Sathyendra V, Darowish M. Basic science of bone healing. *Hand Clin.* 2013 Nov;29(4):473–481.

CHAPTER 2
Emergency management of facial trauma

Current concepts in trauma care

Facial injuries are usually seen in isolation but they are also commonly associated with other injuries, both above and below the clavicle. As such, their management should never be considered in isolation, especially when other injuries may be present or are clearly evident. Generally speaking they are rarely life-threatening, and therefore most facial injuries can safely wait for assessment and management while more serious injuries elsewhere on the patient are being evaluated and treated. However, some facial injuries can be immediately life-threatening, or can become life-threatening over a period of minutes or hours. The two common causes of this are progressive airway obstruction and ongoing haemorrhage, both of which may be overlooked when the patient first arrives in the emergency department. In many trauma victims the mechanism of injury may provide useful clues as to the possibility of hidden or 'occult' injuries, some of which may result in life-threatening problems (Fig. 2.1).

The modern management of trauma is based on a firm understanding of the pathophysiology of trauma and an understanding of how patients actually die. This understanding has led to the development of several trauma systems, of which the Advanced Trauma Life Support (ATLS) is now generally recognized as the 'gold standard'. ATLS was originally introduced by the American College of Surgeons Committee of Trauma and is now taught in over 50 countries worldwide. It provides a systematic approach that should ensure that life-threatening and subsequent injuries are identified and managed in an appropriate and timely manner. Management is based on a number of well-established principles (Table 2.1).

Patient assessment commences with a rapid primary survey (Table 2.2) during which life-saving interventions are undertaken. Urgent investigations and other interventions are then performed. The patient is then re-evaluated (secondary survey), stabilized and when required, transferred to a facility for specialized care. It is during the rapid primary survey that consideration of life-threatening complications of facial injuries should be made.

The importance of the mechanism of injury

An accurate history and understanding of the mechanism of injury is helpful in both general and specific trauma care. In general trauma it may help in the anticipation of occult injuries, such as damage to the spinal cord or internal bleeding not immediately evident. Up to 15% of all injuries have been reported to go the following initial assessment. Delayed onset of life-threatening complications is of particular concern when inter-hospital transfers are being considered. Stabilization prior to transfer may involve a search for specific injuries, based almost entirely on the pattern of injury. Some serious injuries may not be immediately apparent and can take hours, or even days to become clinically detectable. Clinical examination of the chest and abdomen is now generally accepted as unreliable in the trauma setting. For all these reasons an active clinical search for life-threatening injuries together with general body imaging is now frequently undertaken based on the mechanism of injury.

Although not life-threatening, the mechanism of injury will often determine the pattern and displacement of facial bone fractures and injuries to the dentition. Rare penetrating injuries of the periorbita or soft palate may involve the cranial cavity. Missile injuries to the mandible can cause widespread transverse subgingival root fracture of adjacent teeth.

Fractures of the Facial Skeleton, Second Edition. Michael Perry, Andrew Brown and Peter Banks.
© 2015 John Wiley & Sons, Ltd. Published 2015 by John Wiley & Sons, Ltd.

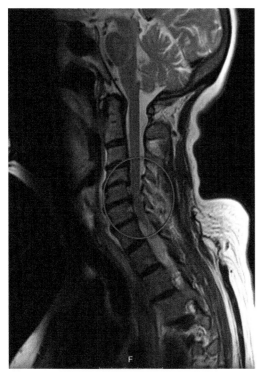

Figure 2.1 MR scan of an elderly female patient taken five days after falling onto her face. In addition to the facial injuries there was also some mild weakness in the right hand. MRI confirmed a central cord syndrome. The clue is the mechanism of injury that resulted in hyperextension of the neck. (Reproduced with kind permission of Springer Science+Business Media.)

Table 2.1 Principles of ATLS management.

ABCDE of assessment (see Table 2.2)
Primum non nocere (First, do no harm)
Concept of the 'golden hour' (i.e. time is of the essence)
Need for frequent reassessment for evolving injuries
Importance of understanding the mechanism of injury

Table 2.2 Rapid primary survey in order of priority.

Airway with cervical spine control
Breathing and ventilation (oxygenation)
Circulation and control of haemorrhage
Disability – assessment of neurological deficit
Exposure and environmental control

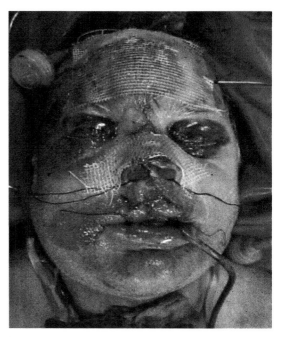

Figure 2.2 Patient with severe facial injury resulting in multiple facial fractures. Extensive swelling develops rapidly within the first few hours. In addition the periorbital haematoma and deformity due to disruption of the naso-orbito-ethmoid complex is obvious. Close monitoring of the airway is essential to detect the onset of possible obstruction. (Reproduced with kind permission of Springer Science+Business Media.)

The multiply injured patient with facial injuries

In the multiply injured patient injuries to the face can vary widely, from the most trivial to those associated with immediate life-threatening complications. To complicate matters, life-threatening complications in facial trauma can develop slowly over a period of several hours, for example airway obstruction from progressive swelling (Fig. 2.2). Facial bleeding can also go unrecognized, especially in supine patients. In some injuries, sight-threatening complications may also occur and these may not be immediately obvious. Initial assessment and management can therefore be very challenging, since all these variables need to be taken into account.

The presence of facial injuries, even minor facial injuries, can have a significant influence on the overall management of the multiply injured patient. For example, a facial injury may mean that the airway needs

Table 2.3 Triaging of facial injuries.

Group	Treatment priority	Example
1	'Within a few seconds'	Immediate life or sight-saving intervention is required – such as establishment of a surgical airway, control of profuse haemorrhage, or lateral canthotomy and cantholysis.
2	'Within a few hours'	Clinically 'urgent' injuries, such as heavily contaminated wounds and some contaminated open fractures (especially skull fractures with exposed dura). The patient is otherwise clinically stable.
3	'Within a few days'	Treatment can wait 24 h if necessary – some compound fractures and most clean lacerations.
4	'Within a week'	Treatment can wait over 24 h if necessary – many simple or closed fractures.

to be protected, if necessary by intubation, before CT scanning. In the same way associated general injuries may compromise the ideal management of the facial injury. Severe general injuries may be of such priority that any definitive management of facial trauma, other than control of bleeding will of necessity have to be postponed.

A team approach is therefore of vital importance, particularly in the early stages of management, when the clinical status of the patient is often most dynamic. To facilitate this team approach most emergency departments now follow locally agreed protocols for the assessment and treatment of the multiply injured patient. Where these are in place they should obviously be followed by facial trauma surgeons, as an integral part of the trauma team.

Facial injuries can broadly be placed into one of four groups, based on the urgency of treatment they require (Table 2.3). Although true maxillofacial and ophthalmic emergencies that require immediate identification and/or management to preserve life or sight are uncommon, it is nevertheless important to be aware that delayed presentation can still occur. Life- and sight-threatening problems can also develop following apparently minor injuries and may be easily overlooked. Because some problems may take a while to become clinically apparent anticipation is the key to good management. It is therefore important to be aware of such early warning signs as snoring, repeated requests to sit up, agitation or persistent tachycardia. Continual reassessment is an important part of patient care and helps to identify these problems early.

Management of facial injuries in the multiply injured patient

Definitive repair of a facial fracture is never a life-saving measure. Initial treatment should only be directed to the patient's general condition. From a maxillofacial perspective immediate intervention is only required if there are problems with:
1 Airway management.
2 Profuse facial bleeding.
3 Sight or vision-threatening injuries.

Of course, head injuries also clearly fall within this context but these require the expertise of a neurosurgeon. Although the specific management of head injuries will not be discussed in detail here, an awareness and understanding of their pathophysiology, diagnosis and management is essential to all trauma physicians.

If no life- or vision-threatening injuries to the face are present, detailed assessment of most facial trauma can wait until comprehensive assessment of the entire patient has been completed. All injuries, both above and below the clavicles, need to be rapidly recognized, prioritized and then managed in a timely and coordinated manner.

Unfortunately clinical circumstances can change suddenly, as injuries or other events evolve and become clinically apparent. These could include for instance, development of signs of a compartment syndrome, a falling level of consciousness or unexpected vomiting. Therefore, as with all forms of trauma, assessment needs to be both systematic and repeated, with anticipation of potential complications before they develop. This is especially pertinent to the face.

Airway management

Whatever the cause, obstruction of the patient's airway will rapidly lead to asphyxia and is therefore the clinician's first concern. The most important factor controlling the patency of the airway in a patient with facial injuries is the level of consciousness. A fully conscious and upright patient is usually able to maintain an adequate airway even in the presence of severe disruption of the facial skeleton. However, a semi- or unconscious patient will rapidly obstruct from the presence of blood and mucus in the airway, inability to cough or inability to adopt a posture to keep the airway clear. Progressive swelling will compound all these problems.

In multiply injured patients, spinal immobilization is initially required owing to concerns regarding possible spinal injuries. This results in an immediate risk to the airway in almost all patients with significant facial injuries. In most conscious patients' blood and secretions are simply swallowed. However, when midface or mandibular fractures are present, swallowing may become painful and ineffective. Early signs of impending obstruction may not be recognized at first, particularly in intoxicated patients or those with associated brain injury. These patients are at a high risk of vomiting and loss of protective airway reflexes. Early endotracheal intubation should therefore be considered in all supine restrained patients with significant facial injuries.

Even relatively minor injuries such as intraoral bleeding, fractures of the teeth or broken dentures can lead to airway obstruction in a semi-conscious patient. Accordingly, the most important initial measures are the clearing of blood and mucus from the mouth and nasopharynx. Suctioning of the pharynx should be undertaken carefully in awake patients. Stimulation of the soft palate and pharynx can trigger vomiting. Alternatively, and only if other injuries permit, placing a patient on his or her side may assist in free drainage.

During the initial assessment of the airway the cervical spine should also be immobilized, either manually by an assistant, or by using a hard collar, blocks and straps. On occasion patients with facial injuries may repeatedly request or attempt to sit up. This goes against ATLS principles, which requires multiply injured patients to be transferred and assessed whilst supine on a spine board. Management of such patients can be very difficult. If the patient becomes combative they may only tolerate a hard collar. Forceful restraint should be avoided, as holding the head simply creates a fulcrum with leverage on the neck as the rest of the body moves. In such cases formal anaesthesia with intubation and ventilation must be considered.

The effects of facial fractures and swelling of the soft tissues of the airway

Contrary to popular belief it is rare for the upper jaw to be pushed significantly downwards and backwards along the inclined skull base as a result of injury. Flattening or 'dishing' of the face results mainly from comminution of the thin bones of the anterior facial skeleton following severe impact. In such an event there is usually considerable bleeding from the nose and nasopharynx and the face will swell rapidly. The attendant degree of head injury may also be quite serious. It is a combination of these factors that threatens to asphyxiate the patient, rather than physical obstruction from displacement of the facial skeleton as a whole. In severe injuries to the nasal complex the nares are blocked with blood clot or may bleed profusely. Any arrest of nasal haemorrhage by anterior or posterior nasal packing can cause complete occlusion.

In the mandible loss of tongue support and significant swelling of the floor of the mouth may occur in patients with displaced bilateral ('bucket handle') or comminuted fractures of the mandible (Fig. 2.3). These tend to follow relatively localized, but high energy impacts. In alert patients self-protection of the airway may still be possible, even if they are supine. However, in the presence of coexisting head injuries or intoxication, loss of tongue control and other protective reflexes may rapidly become a problem. Comminuted fractures of the mandible carry a significant risk to the airway, not only from loss of tongue support, but also from significant soft tissue swelling and intra-oral bleeding. Anaesthesia and intubation should therefore be considered early.

When both midface fractures and mandibular fractures occur at the same time there is a high risk of airway compromise. These injuries emphasize the need for regular assessments. Airway obstruction, unexpected vomiting and hypovolaemia from unrecognized bleeding are all common consequences. Significant soft tissue swelling inevitably occurs and often necessitates prolonged intubation or planned elective tracheostomy. Swelling is common in all facial trauma but it can be unpredictable. Significant swelling can occur in the absence of fractures, notably in patients taking anticoagulants and the elderly. Usually it is the mechanism of injury and the energy transfer involved, not necessarily the fracture pattern, which is most reliable in predicting swelling.

Protecting the airway

In the presence of obvious midface or mandibular fractures any hard collar is going to limit assessment and may prevent the patient from keeping their

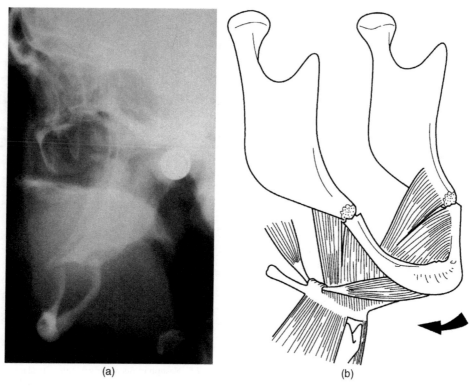

(a) (b)

Figure 2.3 (a) Lateral radiograph showing a bilateral fracture of a very thin mandible with a severe 'bucket handle' type of displacement. (b) Probable mechanism resulting in 'bucket handle' displacement by the suprahyoid musculature. The fracture occurs in the thinnest area of the mandible, anterior to the posterior attachment of the mylohyoid muscle, where bone contact is minimal.

airway clear. This will probably need to be temporarily unfastened to enable initial assessment, but this can be done safely so long as an assistant supports the head. The mouth can then be opened and if required, the mouth and oropharynx cleared. The chin lift and jaw thrust are well known procedures to help improve the airway, but may be difficult to do in a conscious patient with mandibular fractures (Fig. 2.4). They may also aggravate oral bleeding and are usually painful for the patient. A careful examination should be made in case dentures or portions of dentures are still *in situ*. These should be removed together with any avulsed teeth, or loose or broken teeth that are so mobile there is a risk of their being inhaled. Blood and mucus should be cleared using a wide bore blunt-ended pharyngeal sucker. With simple anterior mandibular fractures, if time permits, temporary reduction and stabilization may be possible by placing a 'bridle wire' around the necks of stable teeth either side of the fracture. This can usually be

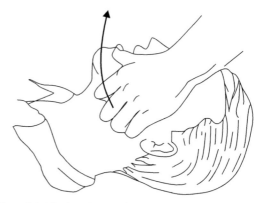

Figure 2.4 The jaw thrust technique used to improve the airway in supine patients. The fingers are placed behind the angle of the mandible to push the jaw forwards and upwards while the thumbs push down on the chin or lower lip to open the mouth. Displacement of the mandible pulls the tongue forward and prevents occlusion of the oro-pharynx. In patients where there is no concern about any cervical injury the neck can be extended and the chin lifted to attain the same end. (John Wiseman, 1986.)

done under local anaesthesia. Reducing the fracture slows bleeding from the torn mucosa and enables the patient to swallow more effectively.

All patients are at risk of unexpected vomiting, but those with facial injuries are at greatest risk. A full stomach, alcohol intoxication and brain injuries are factors that predispose to vomiting. Swallowed blood also seems to be a potent stimulus. These are all commonly associated with facial trauma. It is therefore important to identify those patients who are at such a high risk of vomiting and pulmonary aspiration that they should be anaesthetized and intubated to secure the airway before it happens. Fortunately most patients with minor or moderate facial injuries do not vomit or require urgent measures to secure the airway.

Artificial airways are not well tolerated by conscious patients, owing to the stimulus they invoke from contact with the posterior one-third of the tongue and soft palate. Nasopharyngeal airways are better tolerated than oropharyngeal ones, but are generally considered to be contraindicated if there is the possibility of anterior skull base fractures. The risk of inadvertent intracranial positioning is probably much lower than believed but nevertheless, passing semi-rigid tubes through the nasal cavity may still displace fractures of the cribriform plate and possibly tear the dura. If a nasopharyngeal tube is considered appropriate it should be inserted by an experienced operator, as the distorted nasal skeleton may make passage difficult (Fig. 2.5). The patency of the tube must be maintained by periodic aspiration using a plastic disposable suction catheter attached to the end of the suction apparatus. These flexible disposable sucker ends are invaluable for keeping the pharynx clear in facial injuries. They can be inserted either through a nasopharyngeal tube or through the mouth, even in the presence of intermaxillary fixation.

Continuous supervision of the patient is necessary at this stage, either by the surgeon or by an experienced member of the paramedical staff. The patient's lips should be liberally coated with sterile petroleum jelly to prevent them adhering together with blood clot, and so interfering with respiration. This simple measure should be continued throughout treatment because it does much to ensure the comfort of the patient as well as facilitating oral breathing.

High volume suction (using a wide bore pharyngeal sucker) should always be readily available to clear the airway of blood and secretions, taking care not to induce

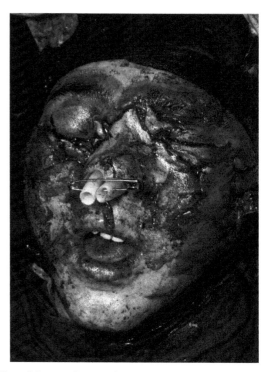

Figure 2.5 Nasopharyngeal airway tubes in place in a patient who has suffered a major facial injury. The ends of the tubes sit behind the tongue base in order to improve upper airway patency but regular aspiration is still mandatory to prevent blockage or pooling of blood and secretions. (Reproduced with kind permission of Springer Science+Business Media.)

vomiting. Loss of the gag reflex during suctioning is an indication for early endotracheal intubation. Although the laryngeal mask airway (LMA) has found widespread use in elective anaesthesia, its emergency use in facial trauma is controversial.

The patient requesting to sit up

Alert patients with facial bone injuries will naturally want to sit up to protect their airway. It is therefore important to recognize the implications of repeated requests, or attempts by a patient to do so.

When injuries to the face have occurred in isolation this posture is permissible. Where possible a hard collar should be applied. However, in the multiply injured patient sitting up will cause an axial load to both the spine and pelvis, potentially displacing any fractures if present. This will occur even if the head is supported. In such cases endotracheal intubation should be considered if the airway is clearly at risk.

The risks and benefits of keeping the patient supine with potential airway obstruction must be weighed against the risks and benefits of axial loading of a possible spinal injury. It follows that a decision to allow a patient to sit up depends on a number of factors that need rapid assessment and careful judgment.

In those patients who cannot sit up or be 'log-rolled' into a safer posture, two critical decisions are therefore necessary. Does the airway need to be secured by anaesthesia and intubation, and if so, how urgently?

Obviously not all patients with facial injuries will develop airway obstruction. Clearly, ability to communicate with the patient is lost once they are anaesthetized and intubated and this will compromise further clinical evaluation; notably assessment of the level of consciousness, abdominal tenderness, spinal assessment and visual acuity. As a result, early intubation often leads to a request for urgent CT scanning of the anaesthetized patient in order to exclude other injuries, which perhaps could have been avoided.

Endotracheal intubation

In the various situations outlined here that may compromise oxygenation the early passage of a definitive airway giving the presence of a cuffed tube in the trachea is by far the most effective way of clearing and preserving the airway.

Intubation may be required if the patient cannot protect their own airway. In addition, if significant swelling is anticipated it is often better to secure the airway early before it becomes too difficult to do so. This requires experienced clinical judgement. If a definitive airway is required urgently the choice includes orotracheal intubation, nasotracheal intubation and surgical cricothyroidotomy.

Endotracheal intubation is also usually required in patients with multiple injuries, particularly combined trauma to the head, face and chest. Occasionally intubation is needed after extensive soft-tissue destruction by a high-velocity missile such as occurs in explosions or military conflict. Generally speaking, rather than carry out an immediate tracheostomy it is preferable to pass an endotracheal tube in the first instance. In a modern intensive care unit a seriously injured patient can be artificially ventilated and monitored for a prolonged period during recovery from multiple injury. Elective tracheostomy should only be considered if and when extubation seems unlikely in the foreseeable future.

Surprisingly, oral endotracheal intubation can be easier than anticipated in patients with extensive fractures. This is because the mobile facial bones can be displaced by the laryngoscope providing an adequate view of the vocal cords. Despite this observation it is nevertheless prudent to be prepared to carry out an immediate surgical airway, just in case airway control is not possible. Difficulty in visualizing the cords is more likely when there is ongoing bleeding and swelling of the pharynx and base of the tongue. Awake fibre-optic intubation, although useful in spinal injuries, is not without risks in the emergency situation with facial injuries since visualization can often be obscured by bleeding. Nasotracheal intubation is regarded by some as potentially dangerous in the presence of anterior cranial base fractures, although this assumption has been strongly challenged in the literature. Ultimately the final choice of technique will probably be made by the anaesthetist.

Emergency surgical airways

The establishment of a surgical airway is occasionally required when the airway cannot be secured by any other means. Members of the trauma team should therefore be competent in performing this procedure if it is urgently required. Emergency surgical airways include needle cricothyroidotomy and surgical cricothyroidotomy (also known as cricothyrotomy).

Needle cricothyroidotomy is a temporary procedure that is sometimes used to oxygenate rapidly patients who are *in extremis* while a definitive airway is being quickly prepared. A cannula is introduced into the lumen of the trachea through the cricothyroid membrane. Oxygen is then delivered by a Y-connector or three-way tap device. However, it is important to note that this procedure will only deliver 250 ml of oxygen into the trachea during each inspiration, some of which will pass into the upper airway rather than down into the lungs. Since the patient is not being ventilated carbon dioxide level control cannot be maintained. A definitive airway should therefore be placed as soon as possible so that the patient can be safely ventilated.

Surgical cricothyroidotomy is now advocated by the American College of Surgeons Committee on Trauma as an appropriate alternative for emergency airway control if endotracheal intubation is not possible. Cricothyroidotomy is an old technique which became discredited because of the apparent risk of sub-glottic stenosis. It is now appreciated that this historical complication

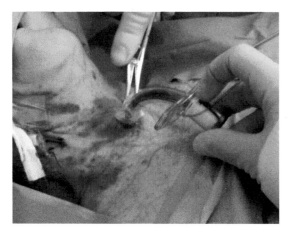

Figure 2.6   Tracheostomy tube being inserted through a cricothyroidotomy incision. Note the use of tracheal dilator forceps to facilitate passage of the slightly smaller than normal tube through the cricothyroid membrane. (Reproduced with kind permission of Springer Science+Business Media.)

Table 2.4 Indications for tracheostomy in maxillofacial injuries.

1 When prolonged artificial ventilation is necessary (for example, associated head and chest injuries).
2 To facilitate anaesthesia during surgical repair of complex facial injuries (consider also submental intubation).
3 To ensure a safe postoperative recovery after extensive surgery.
4 Following obstruction of the airway from laryngeal oedema or occasionally direct injury to the base of the tongue and oropharynx.
5 Following serious haemorrhage into the airway, particularly when a further secondary haemorrhage is a possibility.

usually resulted from performing the operation in children with laryngeal obstruction from infectious diseases. Subsequent studies have shown its efficacy and safety in adults. However, this procedure, which is relatively simple to perform and can be done if necessary under local anaesthesia, is still not appropriate for children or inpatients with inflammation of the trachea.

The key factor in the technique is identification of the cricothyroid membrane. In adults this averages approximately 1 cm vertically and 3 cm horizontally. A slightly smaller tube than usual is therefore required (i.e. cuffed, size 4 or 5). The cricothyroid membrane is usually quite superficial and palpable. The skin and membrane are perforated with a scalpel blade. A standard tracheostomy tube can then be inserted and maintained in the usual manner (Fig. 2.6). Some surgeons prefer to replace a cricothyroidotomy with a tracheostomy within 24 hours. This is because long term cricothyroidotomy stomata have again been reported to be associated with a higher risk of glottic and sub-glottic stenosis than tracheostomies. However, the literature on this is controversial.

Tracheostomy is generally regarded as obsolete in the emergency trauma setting. It is a relatively time-consuming procedure and is potentially unsafe. The trachea is deeper than the cricothyroid membrane and bleeding is more likely if the thyroid isthmus is encountered. For the inexperienced surgeon a surgical cricothyroidotomy is much quicker and safer to perform.

The possible indications for tracheostomy in a patient with maxillofacial injuries are given in Table 2.4.

Breathing problems in facial trauma

In the context of maxillofacial injuries, breathing problems may arise following aspiration of teeth, dentures, vomit and other foreign materials. If teeth or dentures have been lost and the whereabouts are unknown, a chest X-ray and soft tissue views of the neck should be taken to exclude their presence either in the pharynx or lower airway (Fig. 2.7). A plain chest radiograph by itself without neck views is inadequate although this is still common practice. Occasionally CT scanning or fibre-optic endoscopy may be necessary. Unfortunately acrylic is not very obvious on a radiograph and a careful endoscopic search is necessary to identify and remove denture fragments or other foreign bodies.

Circulation and blood loss in facial trauma
Haemorrhagic shock

The majority of fractures of the facial skeleton are relatively closed injuries. In spite of their sometimes extensive nature, life-threatening haemorrhage is very uncommon and haemorrhagic shock is therefore unusual. If shock is present this should immediately raise the suspicion of other injury. Although life-threatening haemorrhage in facial trauma is rare, clinically significant blood loss has been reported to occur in approximately 10% of 'panfacial' fractures. Blood loss in young children especially can quickly result in hypovolaemia (Fig. 2.8).

Maxillofacial bleeding may not always be obvious. Blood can ooze slowly from soft tissue injuries and fractures, even 'minor' ones such as a broken nose.

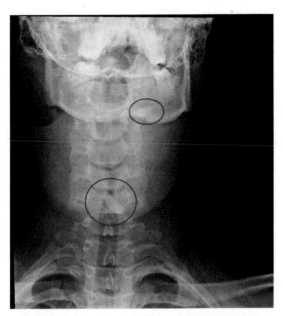

Figure 2.7 Postero-anterior cervical radiograph showing missing avulsed teeth identified in the oro-pharynx and upper trachea. Chest radiographs alone are inadequate when looking for missing teeth in the upper aerodigestive tract. (Reproduced with kind permission of Springer Science+Business Media.)

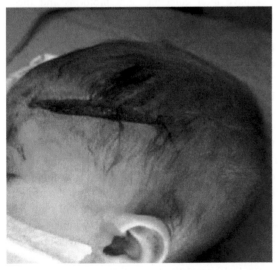

Figure 2.8 Young baby with deep scalp laceration in left fronto-temporal region. Blood loss from maxillofacial injuries in very young patients can be the cause of significant hypovolaemia which should not be underestimated. (Reproduced with kind permission of Springer Science+Business Media.)

Because the blood is often swallowed it is not immediately apparent but a constant trickle over time can become significant. Regular reassessments of the airway should therefore always include a look for fresh blood in the pharynx.

With more severe injuries particularly those with extensive soft-tissue lacerations blood loss can quickly become significant. In these patients bleeding occurs from multiple sites along the fractures and from torn soft tissues, rather than from a single vessel, which makes control difficult. Significant concealed bleeding may occur in any supine patient with facial injuries and should therefore always be considered in cases of persisting shock. These patients are also more likely to develop significant soft tissue swelling and the airway may need to be secured early. Once intubated blood loss then becomes more apparent, as blood is no longer swallowed and overspills from the mouth and nose.

Control of haemorrhage

Significant bleeding from external wounds, such as the scalp, can simply be controlled with pressure or any strong suture to hand. At this stage, the aim is to simply stop the bleeding. A continuous suture is both quick and effective in haemostasis. In the scalp, full thickness 'bites' are required to ensure the vessels are included in the layer. Obvious bleeding vessels should be secured with artery forceps, ligated if possible, and a temporary pressure dressing applied.

Occasionally brisk and persistent haemorrhage originates from a grossly displaced fracture of the mandible or midface. This can only be controlled by manual reduction of the fracture and temporary immobilization either manually, or by means of a wire ligature passed around teeth on each side of the fracture line ('bridle wire'). With very mobile displaced midface fractures, manual reduction may be possible and not only controls blood loss but improves the airway. A well placed mouth prop can sometimes help maintain support. Early intubation should again be considered, not only to protect the airway, but also to allow effective control of bleeding.

Epistaxis

Epistaxis of some degree is an inevitable consequence of injury to the central middle third of the face. This usually stops spontaneously or is easily controlled by lightly packing the nose. Profuse haemorrhage into the nasopharynx may occur rarely in association with a Le Fort type fracture. A postnasal pack is needed in this situation as a matter of urgency. A variety of specifically designed nasal balloons or packs are now widely available. If these specific devices are not available two urinary catheters can be used. Each is passed via both nostrils into the pharynx, inflated with saline and then gently withdrawn until the balloon wedges in the post-nasal space. The nasal cavity can then be packed. Nasal packs are not without risk and aggressive packing should be avoided, especially if anterior cranial fossa or orbital fractures are evident or suspected. Toxic shock, sinusitis, meningitis, brain abscess and even blindness are all rare but potential complications that have been reported. How long packs are left *in situ* will depend on the clinical status of the patient, but around 24–48 hours is usual. If haemorrhage persists despite these interventions it is important to consider coagulation abnormalities that can occur during prolonged resuscitation associated with major blood loss.

Additional surgical control of facial bleeding

Surgical control of facial bleeding is rarely required during the primary survey. Following manual reduction, fractures may be temporarily stabilized using wires, splints, intermaxillary fixation (IMF) or occasionally plating techniques. At this stage the aim is to be quick. Reduction does not need to be anatomical; rather it needs to be sufficient enough to stop the bleeding. External fixation is also very effective in providing rapid 'first aid' stabilization in the multiply injured patient. If bleeding continues despite all these measures, and there are no clotting abnormalities, further interventions include ligation of the external carotid and ethmoidal arteries via the neck and orbit respectively. These steps are rarely required nowadays and are extremely difficult to undertake as emergency procedures. Due to the extensive collateral circulation of the face ligating a single vessel is unlikely to be successful. Add to this the urgency of haemostasis and the fact that the cervical spine may not have been 'cleared', thereby preventing turning of the head for access, and it is little wonder that these techniques are now rarely undertaken. Endovascular radiological intervention, as discussed next, is now the preferred approach.

Superselective embolization

The use of superselective embolization in trauma continues to evolve. It has been extensively reported as very successful, with clear advantages over surgery. It is increasingly used in solid organ and extremity trauma, and in bleeding secondary to pelvic fractures. It is now well documented as a successful treatment modality in penetrating injuries, blunt injuries and intractable epistaxis. Catheter-guided angiography is used to first identify and then occlude the bleeding point(s). Embolization involves the use of a number of materials designed to stimulate clotting locally. Superselective embolization can be performed without the need for a general anaesthetic and in experienced hands is relatively quick. Its value therefore is seen in the unstable patient. Multiple bleeding points can be precisely identified and the technique is repeatable. However, immediate access to specialized radiological facilities and on-site expertise is required.

Disability (associated head injuries in facial trauma)

The comprehensive management of intracranial injuries falls outside the scope of this book but is clearly vital in trauma management in general. Maxillofacial surgeons at all levels of experience need to be aware of this and know when to call a neurosurgeon and what information they will require. Many trauma centres now have local guidelines and protocols and these should be followed whenever possible.

'E' for 'eyes' (vision threatening injuries – VTI)

The conventional designation of the letter 'E' during the rapid primary survey stands for 'exposure and environment'. When this stage is reached in the assessment, all life-threatening conditions both above and below the clavicles should have been identified and managed. The patient is then widely exposed and 'log rolled' to look for other signs of injury. It is also important they are kept warm ('environment'). At this time it is appropriate to consider the possibility of limb and sight-threatening conditions. Limb-threatening conditions would normally be quickly identified; however, sight or vision-threatening conditions can be easily overlooked, especially if the patient has already been intubated. On this basis 'E' is particularly relevant in the presence of facial trauma as a reminder to assess the eyes. Early indications of sight-threatening conditions may also be possible during the disability or 'D' phase of the primary survey when the pupils are assessed.

Although the primary reason for examining the pupils at this stage is to assess for neurological disability, obvious globe injuries will also be noted. Early referral to an ophthalmologist at the appropriate time is then possible. If circumstances and injuries allow a more detailed assessment may be possible once the primary survey is completed using simple instruments and visual acuity charts, but this examination should never interfere with life-saving investigations and interventions. In some respects the assessment of the eyes is similar to the initial assessment of the abdomen and chest during the primary survey. The aim is rapidly to exclude any VTIs in the same way that it is to exclude life-threatening conditions of the abdomen or chest, both of which will require urgent treatment. A precise diagnosis of the injuries at this stage is not important and will be made later, once the patient is stabilized. Early recognition of VTIs in the multiply injured patient is therefore initially based on the mechanism of injury, a high index of suspicion and gross clinical findings, rather than on detailed evaluation which will need to be carried out later. In an awake patient it only takes a few seconds to assess the vision in each eye, check the pupil size and reaction and look for proptosis. The ability to protect the globe, which depends on eyelid integrity, can also be quickly noted. However, visual assessment in the semi-conscious or unconscious patient is extremely difficult and in these patients early diagnosis of eye problems may be easily overlooked or delayed. Apart from the eye response which forms part of the Glasgow Coma Scale estimation (see Appendix at the end of this chapter) clinical assessment in an unconscious patient is basically limited to the evaluation of the pupil size, reaction to light and globe tension on gentle palpation and noting if there is any proptosis.

The presence of a relative afferent pupillary defect (RAPD) is extremely significant. This is tested for by shining a bright light alternately into the left and right eyes. A normal response produces equal constriction of both pupils regardless of which eye the light is directed at, confirming an intact direct and consensual pupillary light reflex. When light is shone into an eye with an RAPD due to optic nerve damage there will be only mild or no constriction of both pupils due to loss of the pupillary reflexes. However, light shone in the unaffected eye will cause a normal constriction of both pupils due to an intact consensual response. In general terms, a brisk reaction to direct and consensual light

Table 2.5 Causes of traumatic loss of vision.

1 Direct injury to the globe.
2 Direct injury to the optic nerve (e.g. bony impingement).
3 Indirect injury to the optic nerve (e.g. deceleration injury resulting in shearing or stretching forces).
4 Generalized or regional fall in tissue perfusion (e.g. anterior ischaemic optic neuropathy, retrobulbar haemorrhage, nutrient vessel disruption).
5 Loss of eyelid integrity.

Table 2.6 Vision threatening injuries in facial trauma.

1 Orbital compartment syndrome and retrobulbar haemorrhage.
2 Traumatic optic neuropathy.
3 Open and closed globe injuries.
4 Loss of eyelid integrity.

stimuli with a round concentric pupil can be regarded as reliable in excluding a VTI requiring immediate intervention.

Possible reasons for a traumatic loss of vision are summarized in Table 2.5, with the more common causes associated with facial trauma shown in Table 2.6 and discussed further later.

Any patient requiring a brain CT, who has suspected periorbital or ocular injuries, should ideally undergo imaging of at least the orbits, and ideally the rest of the face, at the same time. Additional scanning times for this are now negligible (see Chapter 4). Problems such as globe rupture, optic nerve transection, intra-ocular haemorrhage, intra-ocular foreign bodies, periorbital and orbital apex fractures and the nature of any proptosis will all be readily identifiable.

The acutely proptosed eye
Some degree of proptosis following trauma is common and has been reported to occur in approximately 3% of midface injuries. However, *vision-threatening* proptosis is a much rarer event. Critically, retrobulbar pressures that risk causing optic nerve ischaemia need to be recognized early and treated promptly. Irreversible ischaemia of the visual pathway in the orbit can occur within 1 hour, and permanent visual loss within 1½–2 hours. Acute proptosis is usually apparent by the time the patient arrives in the emergency department and unfortunately therefore treatment is often started too late.

Proptosis following trauma can be due to a number of causes, including bony displacement, bleeding, oedema, brain herniation, emphysema, carotid-cavernous fistula and extravasation of radiographic contrast material. Each of these will require different management. However, of all these different causes, oedema (orbital compartment syndrome) is probably the most likely. Retrobulbar haemorrhage is often considered to be a likely cause but in reality is almost certainly much less common than is generally supposed (Fig. 2.9). Whatever the cause, the 'final common pathway' leading to blindness is ischaemia. Since the treatment required in each case varies, one of the most important differentiations to make is between retrobulbar *haemorrhage* (which may need evacuation) and retrobulbar *oedema* (which may resolve medically, or require a different surgical procedure). Urgent treatment of the proptosed globe is therefore extremely difficult, especially if appropriate imaging is unavailable.

The options for management of vision threatening acute proptosis in the resuscitation room are limited. Medical treatments and a lateral canthotomy may 'buy time' while preparing the patient for surgery. Mannitol (1 g per kg) and acetazolamide (250–500 mg) are frequently prescribed, but may be contraindicated in the presence of hypovolaemic shock. High dose steroids are also recommended, but these are considered to be contraindicated if the patient has coexisting severe head injuries. While both lateral canthotomy and cantholysis have been advocated in the medical literature the anatomy and techniques to be used are variably described. Acute proptosis is rare in practice and there are few clinicians who could claim to be experienced in its management.

Whether or not to undertake formal decompression or evacuate a haematoma depends on many things; such as the general condition of the patient, the precise diagnosis of the cause of proptosis, the surgical skills available and the likelihood of salvaging vision. If the patient is awake the state of vision in the affected eye is a good clinical guide, but of course the decision becomes much harder in the unconscious patient. Generally speaking unless treatment is commenced very early the prognosis is poor.

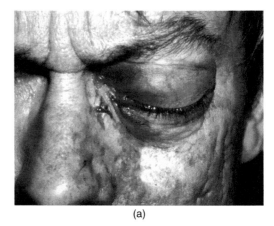

(a)

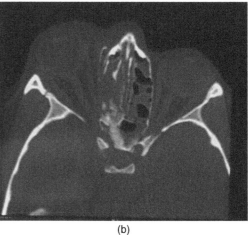

(b)

Figure 2.9 (a) Proptosis of the left eye following an orbital fracture. (b) Axial CT scan of the orbits showing significant anterior displacement of the globe. Not all cases of proptosis following trauma are due to retrobulbar haemorrhage. Many result from retrobulbar oedema, sometimes referred to as 'orbital compartment syndrome'. (Reproduced with kind permission of Springer Science+Business Media.)

Traumatic optic neuropathy

Interestingly, the ancient Greek physician Hippocrates (c. 460–370 BC) noted an association between blunt forehead trauma and blindness which could occur even in the absence of fractures, and is therefore possibly the first to describe traumatic optic neuropathy. The condition occurs in approximately 0.5% of closed head injuries and in some cases the injuring mechanism can be relatively trivial. Following blunt trauma, stretching, contusion or shearing forces can injure the optic nerve as it passes through the bony canal into the orbit. Displaced fractures around the orbital apex can also compress the nerve.

The diagnosis of traumatic optic neuropathy is a clinical one. Visual loss is usually profound and almost instantaneous, but it can be more moderate and delayed. Visual loss is permanent in approximately half of patients affected. A relative afferent pupillary defect is present. Treatment remains controversial and may be medical or surgical. The role for high-dose intravenous corticosteroids is still unclear and may be contraindicated in some patients. The role of surgical decompression is even more controversial.

Open and closed globe injuries

The term 'open globe injury' refers to a full thickness wound in the wall of the eye. This may be caused by blunt trauma causing globe rupture, or by a sharp object producing a penetrating or perforating laceration. A 'closed' globe injury does not result in a full thickness wound and includes superficial foreign bodies and contusions. The possibility of an intraocular foreign body should always be considered, especially if it may be metallic and the patient might require an MRI scan to evaluate other injuries. Important signs of a globe injury that may be immediately apparent are shown in Table 2.7.

Management of a globe injury depends on whether it is open or closed. Analgesia and anti-emetics should be administered and the anti-tetanus status checked. A hard plastic shield should be taped over the eye to protect open injuries. Primary surgical repair of an open globe should ideally be performed within 24 hours. Closed globe injuries are managed with steroid, antibiotic, cycloplegic (ciliary muscle paralysing) and anti-hypertensive eye drops. Generally speaking, an initial poor visual acuity, presence of a relative afferent pupillary defect and posterior involvement of the eye, carry a bad prognosis in both closed and open globe injuries.

Loss of eyelid integrity

Inability to close the eyelids effectively can result rapidly in loss of sight. Even relatively minor eyelid lacerations may predispose to this and may be easily overlooked. Avulsion of the eyelids is a rare but devastating injury and extremely difficult to reconstruct. Eyelid lacerations may also indicate serious underlying ocular injury. Until the defect is repaired, any eyelid remnants should be pulled over to provide corneal cover, if necessary using a suture to achieve this. Liberal application of chloramphenicol or 'artificial tears' ointment should be administered and the whole area covered with a sterile wet gauze swab. If a delay in repair is expected the wound should at least be cleaned and superficial foreign bodies removed. Copious amounts of saline irrigation under light pressure can be used to wash out foreign bodies and reduce the microbial load. Intravenous antibiotic cover is needed for all bite injuries and contaminated wounds. The anti-tetanus status should also be checked.

Further reading

Allen M, Perry M, Burns F. When is a retrobulbar haemorrhage not a retrobulbar haemorrhage? *Int J Oral Maxillofac Surg.* 2010;39:1045–1049.

American Society of Anesthesiologists. Practice guidelines for the management of the difficult airway: a A report by the American Society of Anesthesiologists Task Force on Management of the Difficult Airway. *Anesthesiology.* 1993;78:597–602.

Beuran M, Iordache FM. Damage control surgery: new concept or re-enacting of a classical idea [review]? *J Med Life.* 2008;1:247–253.

Cooper DJ, Ackland HM. Clearing the cervical spine in unconscious head injured patients: the evidence. *Crit Care Resusc.* 2005;7:181–184.

De Waele JJ, Vermassen FE. Coagulopathy, hypothermia and acidosis in trauma patients: the rationale for damage control surgery [review]. *Acta Chir Belg.* 2002;102:313–316.

Table 2.7 Signs of globe injury.

1 Corneal abrasion
2 Hyphaema.
3 Irregular pupil.
4 Prolapsed uvea.
5 Obvious open wound.
6 Collapsed or severely distorted globe.
7 Loss or impairment of the red reflex (the reddish reflection from the retina noted when using an ophthalmoscope from approximately 30 cm).
8 Blood-stained tears.

DiGiacomo C, Neshat KK, Angus LD, Penna K, Sadoff RS, Shaftan GW. Emergency cricothyrotomy. *Mil Med.* 2003;168:541–544.

Perry M. Acute proptosis in trauma: retrobulbar hemorrhage or orbital compartment syndrome: does it really matter? *J Oral Maxillofac Surg.* 2008a;66:1913–1920.

Perry M. Advanced Trauma Life Support (ATLS) and facial trauma: can one size fit all? Part 1. Dilemmas in the management of the multiply injured patient with coexisting facial injuries. *Int J Oral Maxillofac Surg* 2008b;37:209–214.

Perry M, Morris C. Advanced trauma life support (ATLS) and facial trauma: can one size fit all? Part 2: ATLS, maxillofacial injuries and airway management dilemmas. *Int J Oral Maxillofac Surg.* 2008;37:309–320.

Perry M, Moutray T. Advanced Trauma Life Support (ATLS) and facial trauma: can one size fit all? Part 4: 'Can the patient see?' Timely diagnosis, dilemmas and pitfalls in the multiply injured, poorly responsive/unresponsive patient. *Int J Oral Maxillofac Surg.* 2008;37:505–514.

Perry M, O'Hare J, Porter G. Advanced Trauma Life Support (ATLS) and facial trauma: can one size fit all? Part 3: Hypovolaemia and facial injuries in the multiply injured patient. *Int J Oral Maxillofac Surg.* 2008;37:405–414.

Perry M, Moutray T. Advanced Trauma Life Support (ATLS) and facial trauma: can one size fit all? Part 4: 'Can the patient see?' Timely diagnosis, dilemmas and pitfalls in the multiply injured, poorly responsive/ unresponsive patient. *Int J Oral Maxillofac Surg.* 2008;37:505–14.

Appendix

The Glasgow Coma Scale

The Glasgow Coma Scale (GCS) is a method of neurological assessment that provides a reliable, objective way of recording the conscious state of a patient. It can be used for initial evaluation as well as regularly recording improving or deteriorating status. Points are awarded using the criteria given in the scale to give a total score between 3 (deeply unconscious and unresponsive) and 15 (fully conscious, alert and orientated). Any patient with a GCS score of less than 8 should be considered as unable to protect their airway.

	Best motor response (M)		*Best verbal response (V)*		*Best eye response (E)*
1	Makes no movements.	1	No verbal response.	1	No eye opening.
2	Extension to pain – abduction of arm, external rotation of shoulder, supination of forearm, extension of wrist. (Decerebrate response.)	2	Incomprehensible sounds – moaning but no words.	2	Eye opening in response to painful stimulus – fingernail bed pressure, supraorbital or sternal pressure.
3	Abnormal flexion to pain – adduction of arm, internal rotation of shoulder, pronation of forearm, flexion of wrist. (Decorticate response.)	3	Inappropriate words – random speech but no conversation.	3	Eye opening in response to command.
4	Flexion/withdrawal to pain – flexion of elbow, supination of forearm, flexion of wrist when supraorbital pressure applied, pulls part of body away when nail bed pinched.	4	Confused conversation – response to questions but some disorientation and confusion.	4	Spontaneous eye opening.
5	Localizes to pain – purposeful movements towards painful stimuli (e.g. hand crosses mid-line and gets above clavicle when supraorbital pressure applied).	5	Orientated – coherent and appropriate response to questions.		
6	Obeys commands – patient carries out simple requests.				

CHAPTER 3
Clinical features of facial fractures

The clinical features of fractures of the various bones that make up the facial skeleton relate to the surgical anatomy of the face. It is therefore appropriate to review the surgical anatomy, the classification of fracture patterns and the resulting clinical features before moving on to the methods of treatment.

The 'simplest' bony injury is that associated with dental trauma; the dentoalveolar fracture. This injury is discussed separately in Chapter 5.

Fractures of the mandible

Fractures of the mandible are common yet, despite considerable collective experience and extensive literature on the subject, some aspects of care still remain controversial (e.g. management of fractures of the condyle and fractures in severely atrophic jaws). For a number of reasons there are still suboptimal outcomes although the incidence of complications such as infection and malunion has decreased markedly with modern techniques.

Surgical anatomy

Although the mandible is embryologically a membranous bone, its physical structure resembles a bent long bone with two articular cartilages and two nutrient arteries. This arch of cortico-cancellous bone projects down and forwards from the base of the skull and constitutes the strongest and most rigid component of the facial skeleton. The two vertical rami are joined together by a horseshoe shaped strut of tooth supporting bone. Each ramus carries two processes: the condyle, which articulates with the glenoid fossa to form the temporomandibular joint, and the coronoid process that receives the insertion of the temporalis muscle. The condylar head is supported on a relatively slender condylar neck – a frequent site for fracture. Anatomically, the lower jaw is divided into a number of areas that also correspond to sites at which fractures usually occur, as shown in Fig. 3.1.

Owing to its prominence, the mandible is more commonly fractured than the bones of the midface. Furthermore, unlike the 'matchbox-like' midfacial skeleton that readily absorbs direct trauma, blows to the mandible are transmitted directly to the base of the skull through the temporomandibular articulation. This in turn means that relatively minor mandibular fractures may be associated with a surprising degree of closed head injury; hence the effectiveness of the boxer's knock-out punch.

Muscle attachments

The mandible has a number of powerful muscles inserted along its length. These include the muscles of mastication (temporalis, masseter and medial and lateral pterygoids), together with the suprahyoid muscles (digastric, geniohyoid and mylohyoid). Collectively, these muscles control the jaw movements. Some of them can generate considerable biting forces and may play an important role as displacing forces across a fracture. The genioglossus muscle that forms the bulk of the tongue is inserted at the genial tubercles. If the level of consciousness is depressed loss of support for this muscle can place the airway at risk.

Periosteum

The periosteum is a most important structure in determining the stability or otherwise of a mandibular fracture. The periosteum of the mandible is a tough fibrous membrane, and gross displacement of fragments cannot occur if it remains intact and attached to the bone. Periosteum may be stripped from the bone ends by the extremity of the force applied, but

Fractures of the Facial Skeleton, Second Edition. Michael Perry, Andrew Brown and Peter Banks.
© 2015 John Wiley & Sons, Ltd. Published 2015 by John Wiley & Sons, Ltd.

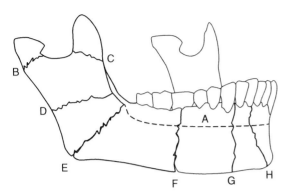

Figure 3.1 Classification of mandibular fracture sites. A dentoalveolar; B condylar; C coronoid; D ramus; E angle; F body (molar/premolar area); G parasymphysis; H symphysis.

more frequently it yields to the accumulation of blood seeping from the ruptured cancellous bone. Once the periosteum has been breached by injury or surgical exposure, displacement and movement of the bones can occur more easily under the influence of the attached muscles.

Teeth

In contrast to the maxilla, tooth sockets in the lower jaw constitute lines of relative weakness and the teeth themselves are a potential source of infection in many mandibular fractures. In its physical structure the mandible resembles a long bone, but a long bone that is subjected to a series of compound fractures each time a tooth is extracted. Such an assault on a limb bone of similar structure, such as the tibia or femur, would lead inevitably to intractable osteomyelitis; whereas in the mandible uneventful healing usually takes place in spite of the wound being bathed in bacteria. The bones of the jaw have developed a special resistance to infection during the course of evolution. The precise mechanism of this is not really understood, although undoubtedly its excellent blood supply and the presence of salivary growth factors play some role. However, any fracture of the mandible with a tooth in the fracture line is nevertheless a compound fracture and the tooth, which may have been devitalized, represents a potential source of infection.

Nerves and blood vessels

On the medial side of the ramus, the inferior alveolar nerve and vessels enter the bone via the mandibular (lingual) foramen, passing forward through the inferior dental canal. These provide sensory innervation and nutrition to the lower teeth. The mental nerve exits the mandible through the mental foramen in the premolar region providing sensory innervation to the lower lip. The inferior dental nerve is vulnerable and frequently damaged when fracture lines cross the inferior dental canal, as occurs in fractures of the body and angle of the mandible. This results in anaesthesia or paraesthesia of the teeth and lower lip.

Branches of the facial nerve lie superficial to the mandibular ramus and are vulnerable to direct trauma to this area. Occasionally the mandibular division of the facial nerve is damaged in association with a fracture of the body or angle.

Injury to major blood vessels is unusual in association with mandibular fractures apart from occasional brisk haemorrhage from the inferior dental vessels. A large sublingual haematoma may result from rupture of dorsal lingual veins in extensive fractures. The facial vessels are also vulnerable to direct trauma where they cross the lower border of the mandible.

Temporomandibular joint

Acute traumatic arthritis can occur as a result of indirectly transmitted violence without there being a fracture of the condyle. A synovial effusion occurs with widening of the joint space on radiographs. The joint is extremely painful and mandibular movement is very restricted.

An intracapsular fracture of the condylar head will frequently cause a haemarthrosis. If this occurs in a young child it can predispose to fibrous or bony ankylosis of the temporomandibular articulation and interference with the growth potential of the condyle.

The meniscus is an important component of the temporomandibular joint. Routine radiographs do not delineate this structure although it can be visualized by magnetic resonance imaging. Nevertheless, knowledge of the incidence of meniscal damage in mandibular trauma remains incomplete. Disruption of the meniscus itself, or the meniscal attachments, may be important in the subsequent function of the joint. There is some evidence that tearing of the meniscus along with haemarthrosis predisposes to late fibrous or bony ankylosis (Fig. 3.2).

Not infrequently a fractured condylar head is driven backwards with sufficient force to tear the lining of the

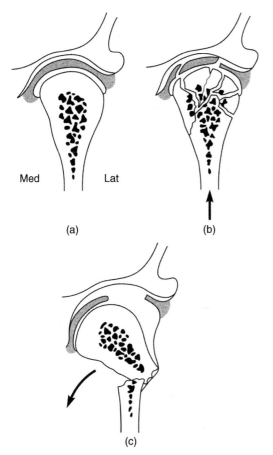

(a)

(b)

(c)

Figure 3.2 Diagrammatic representation of condylar fractures that may cause disruption of the temporomandibular joint meniscus. (a) Coronal view of normal condyle and meniscus. (b) Impaction injury causing intracapsular fracture haemarthrosis and damage to the meniscus. (c) Medial fracture dislocation with tearing of the meniscus.

adjacent external auditory meatus and cause bleeding from the external ear. Such bleeding must be carefully distinguished from middle ear bleeding that signifies a fracture of the base of the skull. Very rarely, the glenoid fossa is fractured as the mandibular condyle is driven against this thin part of the temporal bone. Usually a fracture of the condylar neck prevents this more serious injury occurring.

Mandibular fracture patterns

Cadaveric studies have shown that the impact forces required to produce fractures of the maxilla are considerably lower than those of the mandible (140 lb/65 kg as against 425 lb/190 kg). It is also known that mandibular fracture patterns commonly involve the condylar neck. Fractures of the neck of the condyle can therefore be regarded as a safety mechanism that protects the patient from the serious consequences of a middle cranial fossa fracture. Higher forces still (800–900 lb/350–400 kg) are required to produce fractures of the symphysis and both condylar necks. Studies have also shown that the mandible is much more sensitive to lateral than to frontal impacts presumably due to the fact that frontal impacts at the symphysis are substantially cushioned by opening and retrusion of the jaw or dissipation of forces across the occlusion.

The teeth are important in determining where fractures occur. The long canine tooth and the partially erupted or unerupted wisdom tooth both represent lines of relative weakness (Fig. 3.1 lines G and E). Unerupted teeth such as premolars are important in the same way. The relative frequency of fractures at the recognized sites is as follows:

Condyle	30%
Angle	5%
Body	25%
Symphysis/parasymphysis	15%
Ramus	3%
Coronoid	2%

The alveolar resorption that follows tooth loss also weakens the mandible and fractures of the edentulous body often result from much smaller impact forces. Extreme alveolar resorption can lead to a situation where what is in essence a pathological fracture takes place. Fractures of this nature in a bone perhaps no thicker than a pencil are notoriously difficult to treat.

Mandibular fractures are sometimes described or classified according to their tendency to displace as a result of the pull of the attached muscles (Figs. 3.3 and 3.4). Fractures are said to be 'favourable' when the muscles tend to pull the fragments together (minimizing displacement) and are called 'unfavourable' when they are significantly displaced by the muscles. These are further considered as 'vertically' or 'horizontally' favourable or unfavourable, depending on the direction of displacement. Although this principle can be applied to any fracture of the mandible where there are muscles attached, it is most commonly used with angle fractures.

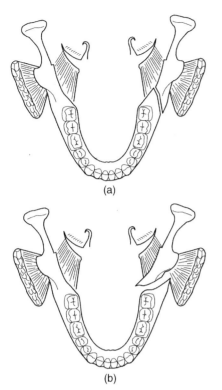

(a)

(b)

Figure 3.3 (a) Vertically favourable and (b) vertically unfavourable fractures of the left angle of the mandible. The classical terminology used here and in Fig. 3.4 is mainly of historical interest. It ignores the stabilizing effect of the periosteum across the fracture line and has little practical relevance now that open reduction and internal fixation is the normal mode of treatment. When mandibular fractures are displaced it is usually as a result of the impact force stripping the periosteum and not muscle pull.

In practice this concept, which was perhaps more relevant when closed reduction was the norm, has little practical value because it ignores the stabilizing effect of the periosteum. It has some importance when the periosteum has been ruptured or stripped from the bone in that a favourable fracture line will make the reduced fragments easier to stabilize.

Fracture of the condylar process

When a fracture of the condylar neck occurs the condylar head is frequently displaced within the articular fossa. This is often, but incorrectly, referred to as a fracture dislocation. The cranio-mandibular articulation is a 'hinge and slide' joint and is not as anatomically stable as a 'ball and socket' joint such as the hip. A so-called 'dislocation'

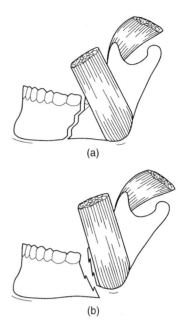

(a)

(b)

Figure 3.4 (a) Horizontally favourable and (b) horizontally unfavourable fractures of the left angle of the mandible. (See caption for Fig. 3.3.)

of the former is more accurately termed a 'subluxation', which fails to reduce spontaneously because of muscle spasm. True dislocation, where the condylar head is displaced completely out of the fossa, is a much rarer event and usually follows significant impacts. The most frequent direction of displacement is medially and forward under the influence of the lateral pterygoid muscle. The importance of this muscle as a displacing force is dramatically illustrated in those cases where anteromedial subluxation occurs some days after injury in a previously undisplaced fracture.

Fractures at the symphysis and parasymphysis

In the symphysis region muscle attachments are important. The mylohyoid muscle constitutes a diaphragm stretching between the hyoid bone and the mylohyoid ridge on the inner aspect of the mandible. In midline fractures of the symphysis the mylohyoid and geniohyoid muscles sometimes act as a stabilizing force. However, an oblique fracture in this region will tend to overlap under the influence of the geniohyoid/mylohyoid diaphragm.

When a bilateral parasymphyseal fracture occurs it usually results from considerable force that disrupts the periosteum over a wide area. Such a fracture is readily displaced posteriorly under the influence of the genioglossus muscle and to a lesser extent, the geniohyoid. It is often stated that such a fracture allows the tongue to fall back and obstruct the oropharynx. This is not in fact the case as the tongue is still firmly attached to the hyoid bone, which in turn remains connected to the mandible by the posterior part of the mylohyoid muscle. In addition, the intrinsic muscles of the tongue continue to exert control and the tongue remains forward in the oral cavity. Voluntary tongue control is only lost when the patient's level of consciousness is depressed, and consequently it is only in these circumstances that the detached symphysis constitutes a threat to the airway (Fig. 3.5). For these reasons supine restrained patients with coexisting head injuries need to be carefully watched.

Fracture of the coronoid process

This is a rare fracture comprising only around 1–2% of all mandibular fractures. It is said to be brought about by reflex muscular contraction of the strong temporalis muscle which then displaces the fragment upwards towards the infratemporal fossa. However, an impact directly onto the side of the face, especially when the mouth is open, can also result in this fracture. Management of isolated coronoid fractures is usually conservative. When the zygomatic arch has also been fractured it is commonly taught that there is a risk of ankylosis between the two healing sites and that surgical treatment is necessary. Being such a rare fracture the evidence for this is entirely anecdotal, although it may appear logical.

Clinical examination

The importance of understanding the mechanism of injury has been discussed elsewhere, and is of particular importance in the mandible. High-energy impacts that are sufficient to break the bone – particularly those resulting in comminuted or multiple-site fractures – not only put patients at risk from cervical spine and head injuries, but can also place the airway at risk from bleeding, swelling and loss of tongue support. High-energy blows to the side of the jaw can also result in significant displacement of fractures involving the inferior dental nerve canal. This in turn may result in traction injuries, or even avulsion of the nerve, adversely affecting the prognosis for functional recovery. The classic 'guardsman's' fracture (i.e. a midline or parasymphyseal fracture, associated with bilateral fractures of the condyles) typically occurs following a faint or fall onto the chin.

The common symptoms and signs of a fractured mandible are summarized in Table 3.1. The hallmark

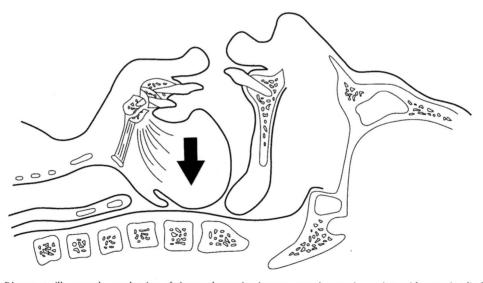

Figure 3.5 Diagram to illustrate the mechanism of airway obstruction in an unconscious supine patient with posterior displacement of the symphysis. This is rarely a problem in a conscious patient even with significant injuries. In this situation the hyoglossus muscle and the intrinsic musculature, aided by the patient's upright posture, will allow control of the airway in almost all cases.

Table 3.1 Common symptoms and signs of mandibular fracture(s).

- Pain: especially on talking and swallowing
- Numbness of the lower lip
- Swelling and drooling
- Trismus and difficulty in moving the jaw
- Bone tenderness over fracture site
- Altered occlusion
- Loosened teeth and gingival bleeding
- Mobility of fractured segment
- Haematoma associated with fracture site, especially sublingual

of a mandibular fracture is a change in the patient's occlusion; an important sign that can be easily overlooked or misinterpreted by the non-specialist.

Condylar fractures

These are the most common fractures of the mandible and are the ones most commonly missed on clinical examination. Condylar fractures may be unilateral or bilateral and they may either involve the joint compartment (intracapsular fractures) or the condylar neck (extracapsular fractures). The latter are the more common. Extracapsular fractures can occur with or without dislocation or subluxation of the condylar head and the upper fragment may either remain angulated compared to the lower portion of the ramus or be displaced medially or laterally. The commonest displacement is antero-medial owing to the direction of pull of the lateral pterygoid muscle that is attached to the antero-medial aspect of the condylar head and also to the meniscus of the temporomandibular joint. In the immediate post-traumatic phase most fractures in the condylar region exhibit similar signs and symptoms. Medial displacement of the condyle can on rare occasions compress the trigeminal nerve. Facial weakness following direct blows to the side of the mandible has also been reported.

Unilateral condylar fractures
Inspection
Any movement of the lower jaw is likely to be restricted and painful. There is often swelling over the temporomandibular joint area and there may be haemorrhage from the ear on that side. Bleeding from the ear results from laceration of the anterior wall of the external auditory meatus, caused by violent movement of the

condylar head against the skin in this region. In the normal subject the close relationship of the condyle to the skin of the external auditory meatus can be appreciated if the little finger is placed within the external ear and the jaw moved.

It is important to distinguish bleeding originating in the external auditory canal from the more serious middle ear haemorrhage. The latter signifies a fracture of the petrous temporal bone and may be accompanied by cerebrospinal otorrhoea. In all cases of suspected condylar fracture the ear should be examined carefully with an otoscope.

Occasionally the haematoma surrounding a fractured condyle may track downwards and backwards below the external auditory canal. This gives rise to ecchymosis of the skin just below the mastoid process on the same side. This particular physical sign also occurs with fractures of the base of the skull, when it is known as 'Battle's sign'. This can potentially result in some diagnostic confusion.

On the extremely rare occasion when the condylar head is impacted through the roof of the glenoid fossa, the mandible may be locked and middle ear bleeding may present externally.

If the condylar head is dislocated medially and the oedema has subsided, it may be possible to observe a characteristic hollow over the region of the condylar head, but in the immediate post-traumatic phase this physical sign is usually obscured by oedema.

Palpation
In the recently injured patient there is invariably tenderness over the condylar area. When post-traumatic oedema is present it is difficult to palpate the condylar head and what is believed to be the condylar head may, in fact, be that portion of the condylar neck continuous with the ramus. It may be possible to determine whether the condylar head is displaced from the glenoid fossa by palpation within the external auditory meatus. Standing in front of the patient both little fingers can be hooked into each external auditory meatus and the position and movement of each condylar head compared.

Intraoral examination
Displacement of the condyle from the fossa, or over-riding of the fractures ('telescoping'), shortens the ramus on the affected side and produces premature contact of the occlusion on the ipsilateral molar teeth (Fig. 3.6). The mandible deviates on opening towards

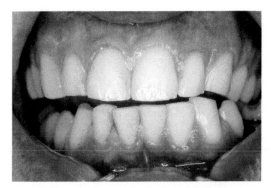

Figure 3.6 Occlusal disturbance produced by a unilateral displaced fracture of the left condylar neck. There is effective shortening of the ipsilateral ramus height leading to premature contact of the molar teeth. Deviation of the mandible to the affected side is also evident.

the side of the fracture and there is usually painful limitation of protrusion and lateral excursion to the opposite side.

Bilateral condylar fractures

The signs and symptoms already mentioned for the unilateral fracture may be present on both sides. Overall mandibular movement is usually more restricted than is the case with a unilateral fracture.

Intraoral examination

Condylar displacement with shortening of the ramus leads to premature contact of the posterior teeth on the side of injury. As would be expected derangement of the occlusion is more usual with bilateral than with unilateral condylar fractures. However, intracapsular fractures produce little if any shortening of ramus height and the occlusion is often found to be normal. If both fractures have resulted in displacement of the condyles from the glenoid fossa, or over-riding of the fractured bone ends, an anterior open bite is found to be present (Fig. 3.7). In all cases of bilateral fracture there is pain and limitation of opening with restricted protrusion and lateral excursions.

Bilateral condylar fractures are frequently associated with fractures of the symphysis or parasymphysis and these areas should always be carefully examined.

Fracture of the angle

In contrast to fractures of the tooth bearing portion of the mandible, the signs and symptoms are not

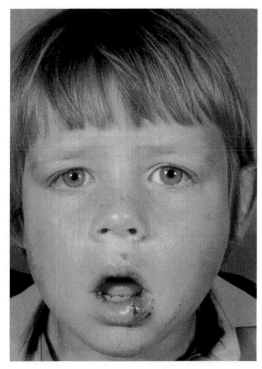

Figure 3.7 A young patient with bilateral displaced condylar neck fractures leading to an anterior open bite. In addition there is swelling over both fracture sites and painful limitation of all jaw movements.

markedly influenced by the degree of displacement of the bone ends.

Inspection

Movements of the mandible are painful and trismus is frequently present to some degree. There is usually swelling at the angle externally and there may be obvious deformity. Within the mouth a step deformity behind the last molar tooth may be visible, which is more apparent if no teeth are present in the molar region. When teeth are present the occlusion is often deranged. Undisplaced fractures are usually detected by the presence of a small haematoma adjacent to the angle on either the lingual or buccal side or both. Anaesthesia or paraesthesia of the lower lip may be present on the side of the fracture

Palpation

There is always bone tenderness on palpation of the angle externally. Movement or crepitus at the fracture site can be felt if the ramus is steadied between finger and thumb and the body of the mandible moved gently with the other hand. A step may be palpated even if it is not evident on inspection.

Fracture of the body (molar and premolar region)

The physical signs and symptoms are similar to those of fractures of the angle as far as swelling and bone tenderness are concerned. In the dentate mandible even slight displacement of the fracture can cause derangement of the occlusion. Premature contact usually occurs on the proximal fragment as a result of the displacing action of the muscles attached to the ramus. Because of the firm gingival attachment, fractures between adjacent teeth tend to cause gingival tears and bleeding. When there is gross displacement, the inferior alveolar neurovascular bundle may be torn and this can give rise to significant intra-oral haemorrhage in addition to anaesthesia or paraesthesia within the distribution of the inferior dental nerve. Altered sensation normally signifies stretching of the inferior alveolar nerve as a result of fracture displacement. Documentation of numbness before any fracture repair is particularly important as any persistence is often a source of patient dissatisfaction and litigation.

Teeth in the fracture line, particularly molar teeth, may be split vertically and cause considerable discomfort if the inferior alveolar nerve remains functional to any degree.

Fractures of the parasymphysis and symphysis

These fractures are commonly associated with fractures of one or both condyles. With minor impacts, the thickness of the anterior mandible between the canine regions often ensures that the fractures are fine cracks that are little displaced and may be missed if the occlusion is undisturbed locally. The presence of bone tenderness and a sublingual haematoma may be the only obvious physical signs (Fig. 3.8).

More severe impact over the symphysis can lead to considerable disruption of the anatomy. A single fracture line is often oblique that allows over-riding of the fragments and lingual inversion of the occlusion on each side. Frequently, trauma to this degree results in bilateral parasymphyseal fractures or comminution of the whole symphyseal bone. There is often associated soft-tissue injury of the chin and lower lip, since these fractures are always caused by direct violence.

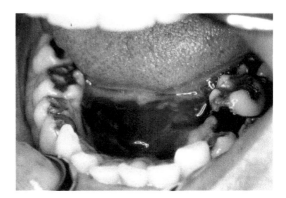

Figure 3.8 Haematoma in floor of mouth as a result of an anterior mandibular fracture. This can be considered as a pathognomic sign of an underlying fracture when there is a clear history of an external blow.

These fracture patterns are often associated with quite severe concussion, in which case the separation of the fragment to which the genioglossus muscle is attached may contribute to loss of voluntary tongue control and obstruction of the airway (Fig. 3.9). If consciousness is not impaired, considerable disorganization of the anterior mandible and the adjacent soft tissue can take place without any significant loss of voluntary control of the tongue (Fig. 3.10).

A fracture of the symphysis is not accompanied by anaesthesia of the skin of the mental region unless the mental nerves are injured after emergence from their foramina.

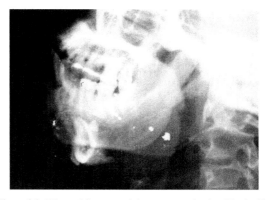

Figure 3.9 Bilateral fracture of the parasymphysis with significant posterior displacement of the anterior mandibular segment. Despite this there was no evidence of airway embarrassment, demonstrating the innate ability of a conscious patient to maintain an airway in most situations. An unconscious supine patient would almost certainly obstruct with this type of injury.

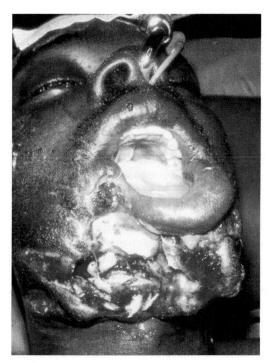

Figure 3.10 Missile injury to the lower face and anterior mandible. Despite the loss of soft and hard tissue, and comminution of the remaining bone, the airway remained intact in this patient who was not rendered unconscious by his injury.

Fracture of the ramus

Fractures confined to the ramus are not common. There are two main types.

1 *Simple (linear) fracture.* This is an uncommon injury and is normally, in effect, a very low condylar fracture running almost vertically downwards from the sigmoid notch. Occasionally as a result of direct violence, a more horizontal linear fracture can occur with both the coronoid and condylar processes on the superior fragment.

2 *Comminuted fracture.* This always results from direct violence to the side of the face. It is a relatively common fracture in missile injuries but is uncommon in civilian practice. The fragments tend to be splinted between the masseter and medial pterygoid muscles and little displacement occurs unless there has been extreme violence.

In both types swelling and ecchymosis is usually noted both extra- and intra-orally. There is tenderness over the ramus and movements produce pain over the same area. Severe trismus is usually present.

Fracture of the coronoid process

This rare fracture is difficult to diagnose clinically but there may be tenderness over the anterior part of the ramus and a tell-tale haematoma. There may be painful limitation of mandibular movement, especially protrusion.

Multiple and comminuted fractures

The physical signs of multiple and comminuted fractures depend on the site and number of the fractures. Multiple and comminuted fractures result from extreme direct violence and are usually associated with severe soft-tissue injury. The precise pattern of bony injury may be impossible to determine from the clinical examination. When there is unexpected mobility of what at first sight appears to be a single fracture, a second fracture on the same side should be suspected. In general comminuted fractures of the ramus, angle and molar regions are not associated with gross displacement of the fragments. However, comminution of the symphysis allows the lateral segments to collapse and presents a much more serious problem of management.

Fractures of the midface and upper face

The midfacial skeleton is a complex anatomical region that can be considered as being composed of several distinct areas. Injuries to each site will have their own structural, aesthetic and functional characteristics and often several sites are involved. Fractures of the tooth bearing part of the midface are variably associated with fractures of the naso-orbito-ethmoid (NOE) region and the zygomatic complex. They may also extend upwards, into the anterior cranial fossa. The bones of the midface are important in the maintenance of the integrity of the oral cavity, nasal cavity and orbits. Not surprisingly, injuries here have significant functional and cosmetic implications. Fractures of the midface tend to result from high-energy impacts and can therefore be both life-threatening as well as disfiguring.

Surgical anatomy
The upper facial skeleton

The so-called 'upper third' of the facial skeleton is chiefly the frontal bone, making up the superior orbital margins and orbital roofs. The base of the skull extends backwards and is angled downwards at approximately 45° where the frontal bone articulates with the sphenoid. The midfacial complex articulates with this sloping plane (see Fig. 3.12). The cribriform plate of the ethmoid extends upwards to make contact with the meninges of the brain and transmits the olfactory nerves (see Fig. 1.4). In cases of predominantly facial trauma the frontal bone and sphenoid are rarely fractured because to a considerable extent they are protected by the cushioning effect of the collapsing weaker bones comprising the midface. When fractures of the cranial component of the facial skeleton occur concomitantly there are important consequences:

1 The brain may have sustained direct injury.
2 The brain may be at risk from indirect injury secondary to bleeding at the fracture site.
3 The fracture may involve the posterior wall of the frontal sinus, the orbital roof, or the cribriform plate, which in turn may be associated with a breach of the dura mater and leakage of cerebrospinal fluid.
4 Displacement, particularly in a caudal direction will interfere with reduction of the facial bones as a whole.
5 Such high energy impacts are frequently associated with cervical spine and ocular and/or optic nerve injuries.

The midfacial skeleton

As previously noted, the composite structure of the complex of bones that forms the 'middle third' of the facial skeleton is so ordered that it is able to withstand the forces of mastication from below and provide protection for vital structures, notably the eyes. Conceptually the midfacial skeleton consists of a series of bone struts passing upwards from the upper teeth to the bone of the skull. The forces of mastication are thus distributed round the fragile area of the nose and paranasal sinuses to the base of the skull. However, the facial bones as a whole have a very low tolerance to impact forces. The nasal bones are least resistant, followed by the zygomatic arch, while the maxilla itself is very sensitive to horizontal impacts. The various bones that make up the midfacial skeleton are listed in Table 3.2.

The Le Fort classification

Fractures of the midfacial skeleton that involve the occlusion of the teeth are invariably multiple as far as the individual bones of the face are concerned. With lower impact energies the general pattern of fracture

Table 3.2 Bones of the midfacial skeleton (see Fig. 1.1).

Two maxillae
Two zygomatic bones
Two zygomatic processes of the temporal bones
Two palatine bones
Two nasal bones
Two lacrimal bones
The vomer
The ethmoid and its attached conchae
Two inferior conchae
The pterygoid plates of the sphenoid

of these bones is remarkably consistent and follows the lines of weakness within the bones of the face described classically by Guérin (1866) and Le Fort (1901). The Le Fort classification of midface fractures (Fig. 3.11) has been used for many years and is well described in many texts but in the modern context is becoming more of historical interest rather than practical value. It was a useful clinical tool when the only way to reduce and immobilize fractures of the midface was to fix a mobilized block of bone to the vault of the skull by some form of external fixation. This took no account of the complexity of the fractures within the block of bone defined by the Le Fort description. Modern CT imaging means that a precise definition and even three-dimensional reconstruction of the fracture pattern is rapidly available in most accident departments. The development of miniature fixation plates and cosmetically acceptable surgical access to the fracture sites now enables accurate primary reconstruction in the majority of cases. Nevertheless, in a broad description of the signs and symptoms of midface fractures the Le Fort terminology is still useful and remains in common use.

Articulation with the base of the skull

If the bones comprising the midfacial skeleton are removed from the skull, it will be seen that the frontal bone and body of the sphenoid form an inclined plane that slopes downwards and backwards from the frontal bone at an angle of about 45° to the occlusal plane of the upper teeth (Fig. 3.12a). The bones of the midfacial skeleton articulate with these strong foundation bones and when fractures occur they are crushed or sheared off the cranial base. The amount of backward displacement is usually only slight but because of

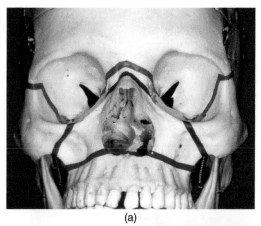

(a)

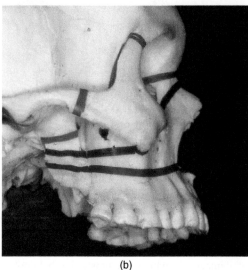

(b)

Figure 3.11 The classical lines of midface fracture as described by Le Fort (a) Frontal view, (b) Lateral view. *Red*: Le Fort I, Guérin or low level transverse fracture. *Blue*: Le Fort II, mid level pyramidal or infra-zygomatic fracture. *Green*: Le Fort III, high level transverse or supra-zygomatic fracture. Although this terminology has a venerable history in the maxillofacial literature modern imaging techniques confirm that injuries are usually considerably more complex than this 'monobloc' pattern suggests.

the steep slope of the base of the skull the posterior teeth of the maxillae contact the posterior mandibular teeth prematurely and produce an anterior open bite (Fig. 3.12b). Occasionally this displacement is sufficient to cause lengthening of the face and in extreme cases the soft palate may be pushed down upon the dorsum of the tongue causing embarrassment to the airway. The situation is compounded by swelling of the soft tissues

and occlusion of the nares by blood clot. It must be remembered that although such physical impairment of the airway is a serious threat to life, a conscious patient will be able to compensate and survive. The real danger to life exists when there is coincident head injury and depression of the level of consciousness in a supine and possibly restrained patient. In this situation the patient will rapidly suffocate unless the airway is protected, or the patient placed in a lateral or prone position.

The facial deformity resulting from disarticulation of the midface from the base of the skull is compounded by collapse of the weaker components of the facial skeleton. The bones of the nasoethmoidal complex and anterior maxillae are particularly affected and it is this inward crushing that produces the characteristic 'dish-face' deformity, rather than total posterior displacement of the whole maxillary complex (Fig. 3.12c).

Involvement of the dura and cranial nerves

Comminution of the ethmoid bones occurs with high level fractures and some severe fractures of the nasal complex. This may be associated with dural tears in the region of the cribriform plate, resulting in cerebrospinal rhinorrhoea. A dural tear may also occur adjacent to fractures involving the posterior wall of the frontal sinus. Cerebrospinal fluid (CSF) may also escape into the soft tissues via coincident fractures of the orbital roof without appearing in the nasal cavity. More rarely, a profuse cerebrospinal rhinorrhoea occurs as a result of a fracture that passes through the sphenoid within the middle cranial fossa.

Clinical detection of CSF rhinorrhoea may be complicated by the presence of lacrimal fluid, blood and nasal secretions. Traditional methods such as testing for glucose or protein are neither sensitive nor specific. Testing the discharge for beta-2 transferrin, a brain specific variant of transferrin, is accepted as the best available diagnostic method. CSF rhinorrhoea is often unilateral (Fig. 3.13).

Damage to the infraorbital and zygomatic nerves may occur with lateral and midface fractures that involve the orbital floor either unilaterally or bilaterally resulting in anaesthesia or paraesthesia of the skin of the cheek and upper lip. The anterior, middle and posterior superior alveolar nerves are also frequently damaged leading to anaesthesia of the upper teeth and gingiva.

The cranial nerves within the orbit may sustain damage in zygomatic and high midface fractures. The sixth

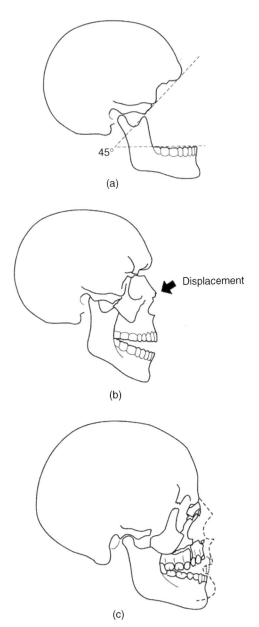

(a)

(b)

Displacement

(c)

Figure 3.12 (a) Diagram to show how the orbital plate of the frontal bone and the sphenoid bone form an inclined plane which lies at approximately 45°to the occlusal plane. (b) In Le Fort II and III type fractures there may be infero-posterior displacement of the midfacial skeleton along this plane resulting in premature contact of the posterior teeth and an anterior open bite. Rarely, with extreme displacement, occlusion of the oral airway can occur due to retroposition of the soft palate. (c) More commonly, the complex of bones is comminuted on impact producing a 'dish-face' deformity with lengthening of the midface. This often gives the impression of greater posterior displacement than has actually occurred.

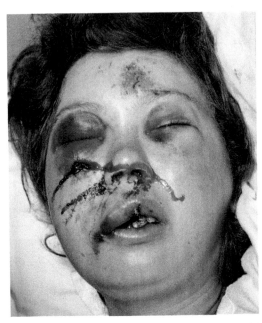

Figure 3.13 Patient with a high level midface fracture involving the cribriform plate with breach of the dura mater and cerebrospinal fluid (CSF) rhinorrhoea. The mixture of CSF (which does not coagulate) and blood (which does) results in a so-called 'tramline' pattern of discharge from the nose, as seen on the patient's left side. Note also the classical signs of a high level fracture including bilateral circumorbital ecchymosis ('panda eyes') and early gross facial swelling.

cranial nerve is most frequently involved resulting in loss of lateral abduction of the eye.

Sometimes the contents of the superior orbital fissure are all damaged, in which case ptosis, ophthalmoplegia and anaesthesia within the distribution of the ophthalmic branch of the fifth cranial nerve are noted (Fig. 3.14). Rarely the orbital apex is fractured with resultant damage to the optic nerve and blindness.

Involvement of the orbit

The globe of the eye and the optic nerve are remarkably well protected by the physical structure and arrangement of the bones of the orbit. The prominence of the zygomatic bone acts as a protection for the globe from all impinging objects other than very small projectiles. The optic foramen is a ring of compact bone and in high level transverse (Le Fort III type) injuries fractures almost invariably pass around it. Rupture of the globe or tearing of the optic nerve is therefore fortunately rarely found with other than the most severe midface fractures.

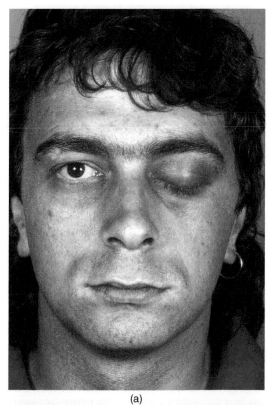

(a)

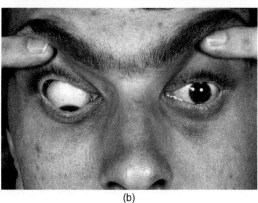

(b)

Figure 3.14 Superior orbital fissure syndrome due to fracture involving the left posterior orbit. (a) Paralysis and ptosis of upper eyelid. (b) Ophthalmoplegia with lack of movement of left eye in all positions of gaze (attempted downward gaze shown here). The patient also had anaesthesia of the left cornea and supra-orbital region. All these signs and symptoms usually resolve spontaneously with time.

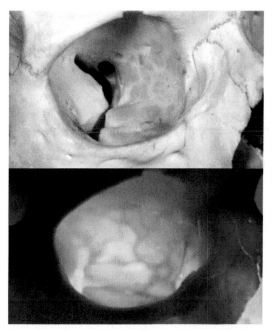

Figure 3.15 Skull transilluminated from behind to show the relative strengths of the orbital bones. The extreme thinness of the floor and medial wall contrasts with the dense bone of the zygoma and orbital rim.

In contrast to the dense ring of bone that comprises the orbital rim, the inferior and medial walls are extremely thin (Fig. 3.15). As a result they are easily fractured allowing orbital contains to herniate through into the maxillary antrum or the ethmoid area. The consequences of this occurring will be discussed in the section on orbital floor fractures later.

Medially sited fractures may involve the nasolacrimal duct with resulting epiphora. This complication is not usually noticed at the time of injury, but may become apparent later.

The paranasal sinuses

In most midface fractures the paranasal sinuses are involved, particularly the maxillary sinus. The thin bony walls are often grossly comminuted with bleeding into the cavity, which results in one or more of the paranasal sinuses appearing opaque on radiological examination. Apart from the routine reduction and repositioning of the fracture, no other special treatment is required and the radiological appearance of the sinuses will return to normal within about 6 weeks.

Uncommonly following a fracture extending into one or other paranasal air sinus air may escape into the soft tissues of the face. This surgical emphysema usually affects the flaccid tissues of the eyelids and gives rise to the physical sign of 'crepitation' of the soft tissues when they are palpated. Whenever air gains entry into soft tissue planes it is contaminated, and adds to the risk of subsequent infection. Air within the cranial cavity or the mediastinum is particularly dangerous. This is a rare complication of facial trauma, but can be seen in patients that have repeatedly and forcefully blown their noses after injury.

Important blood vessels

The third part of the maxillary artery and its terminal branches are closely associated with the lines of fracture of the midface. Occasionally the artery or its greater palatine branch is torn in the region of the pterygomaxillary fissure or pterygopalatine canal resulting in severe haemorrhage into the nasopharynx. Packing of the nose via the anterior nares, whilst usually sufficing in more minor nasal haemorrhage, will be ineffectual in this event and a post-nasal pack or balloon must be inserted. It is necessary to retain this for 24 hours and to replace it if necessary. A pack is a potent source of infection and is not well tolerated by the patient. Adequate reduction of the fracture will fortunately prevent further bleeding in most cases. (See management of epistaxis and control of bleeding pp. 17–18.)

Fractures of the zygomatic complex

Classification

The zygomatic bone is intimately associated with the maxilla, frontal and temporal bones, and since they are also usually involved when a zygomatic bone fracture occurs, it is more accurate to refer to such injuries as 'zygomatic complex fractures'. The descriptive term 'malar fracture' is also sometimes used, malar being the generic word pertaining to the cheek.

The zygomatic complex usually fractures in the region of the frontozygomatic, the zygomaticotemporal and the zygomaticomaxillary sutures (Fig. 3.16). It is unusual for the zygomatic bone itself to be fractured, but occasionally it may be split when there has been extreme violence. Sometimes the bone may even be comminuted.

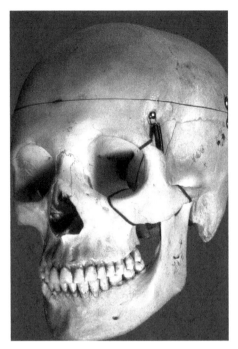

Figure 3.16 Typical zygomatic fracture lines. These rarely coincide exactly with the suture lines of the zygomatic bone, particularly medially, hence the more accurate terms 'zygomatic complex fracture' or 'orbito-zygomatic fracture'. Note the usual proximity of the medial fracture line to the infraorbital foramen that explains the frequent finding of sensory loss over the cheek area and lateral nose.

The arch of the zygoma may be fractured in isolation from the rest of the bone.

Many authors have attempted classification of these injuries. However, these are now mostly historical since modern surgical techniques have rendered management based on their application largely obsolete. Previous classifications attempted to draw inference from either rotation around key landmarks (Rowe and Williams), types of displacement (Knight and North) or patterns of fracture (Jackson). Others have focused on key displacements (e.g. at the frontozygomatic suture: Henderson).

With current imaging and fixation techniques it is perhaps more useful to conceptualize these injuries according to the type and direction of displacement, sites of fractures and degree of comminution; and then to focus upon the surgical approaches and types of fixation required. A simple practical classification is shown in the Table 3.3.

Table 3.3 A practical classification of zygomatic fractures.

Segmental
   a. Zygomatic arch
   b. Infraorbital rim
Minimally displaced
Displaced
Comminuted
   a. Associated with midface or complex orbital fractures
   b. Associated with soft tissue including ocular injury

An understanding of the nature of the displacement of the zygomatic complex is of value when planning the reduction of the fracture and in evaluating the probable stability of the fragments after reduction. When the zygomatic complex is rotated around a vertical axis running through the frontozygomatic suture and first molar tooth, it tends to be stable after simple reduction. However, if displacement occurs round a horizontal axis running through the infraorbital foramen and the zygomatic arch, simple reduction of the fracture is likely to be unstable. In this latter group of fractures there is separation at the frontozygomatic suture. Fractures of the zygomatic complex that are either comminuted, or in which the periosteum of the frontozygomatic suture is torn, are inherently unstable after simple reduction and therefore need fixation.

Signs and symptoms

Since all zygomaticomaxillary fractures by definition involve the orbit, patients should be assessed early for ocular injury, diplopia and entrapment of the orbital soft tissues. The signs and symptoms of a fracture of the zygomatic bone are closely related to the surgical anatomy (see Table 3.4, p. 40).

Flattening of the cheek

When the zygomatic bone is fractured as a block related to its principal three suture lines, it forms a tripod most often displaced inwards to a greater or lesser extent. There may be minimal displacement or an obvious unsightly flattening of the cheek on that side (Fig. 3.17). Tenderness is noted at the fracture lines, particularly over the frontozygomatic suture and an obvious step may be present at the infraorbital margin.

The amount of depression may be masked in a full cheeked individual whereas certain ethnic types with

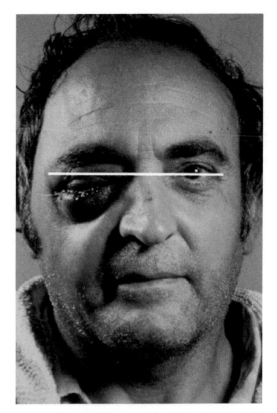

Figure 3.17 Severe orbito-zygomatic injury with periorbital haematoma, flattening of the cheek, vertical separation of the frontozygomatic suture and consequent increase in orbital volume. The resulting enophthalmos, drop in position of the globe (hypoglobus) and pseudoptosis ('hooding') are obvious despite the swelling and haematoma.

prominent cheek bones, may exhibit marked flattening of the face with only moderate inward displacement of the underlying skeleton. The speed with which oedema occurs varies considerably. In some thin, elderly patients, flattening may be obvious up to about an hour after the injury whereas young plump-faced individuals swell up almost immediately. It is always possible to palpate the zygoma at the point of maximum prominence of the cheek. If oedema is masking the flattening, the examiner should view the cheek prominence from above and behind the patient, with each forefinger placed on the point of maximum prominence on each side. The relative position of the tips of the fingers can then be readily compared. Even with marked oedema this manoeuvre enables an assessment to be made of the degree of flattening. Most of the overlying swelling subsides in about a week, but the full extent of the flattening is not apparent until all oedema has completely disappeared, which takes up to 3 weeks.

Haemorrhage

The pattern of haemorrhage around the orbit after injury is so variable that it has little diagnostic value as regards underlying bony injury (Fig. 3.18). Circum-orbital ecchymosis occurs in most cases of zygomatic fracture as well as with central midface fractures. Fractures that involve the orbital walls tend to be accompanied by subconjunctival haemorrhage but its absence in a patient with a 'black eye' does not exclude the presence of a fracture. Ecchymosis of the eyelids alone is usually caused by soft-tissue injury. The extravasated blood is not confined by the orbital septum and spreads wherever the skin is loose, including across the bridge of the nose.

Fractures of the orbital walls may be accompanied by subperiosteal haemorrhage and if the periorbita is damaged this may extend into the conjunctiva. This presents as a 'red eye' where there is bleeding within the conjunctiva with no identifiable posterior limit to the haemorrhage.

Haemorrhage or oedema within the muscle cone of the eye (retrobulbar haemorrhage/oedema) can very

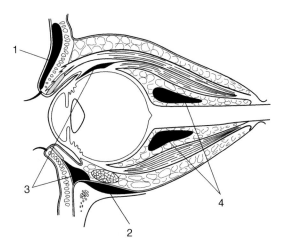

Figure 3.18 Diagram illustrating possible locations of haemorrhage in the orbital area following trauma. 1. Lid ecchymosis. 2. Subperiosteal haematoma. 3. Haemorrhage posterior to the orbital septum (including subconjunctival haemorrhage). 4. Haemorrhage within the muscle cone (retro-bulbar haemorrhage). (Adapted from Soll (1977). Reproduced with permission of American Academy of Ophthamology and Otolaryngology.)

rarely lead to loss of vision. This is thought to occur as a result of spasm of the short posterior ciliary arteries, causing ischaemia of the optic nerve head over a limited but critical area.

When the zygomatic bone is displaced sufficiently, the maxillary antrum fills with blood. This can be seen on plain radiographs as an opacity of the antrum. Following injury and for a short time afterwards, the blood escapes through the antral ostium into the nose and produces a unilateral epistaxis.

Nerve damage

Most fractures of the body of the zygomatic complex involve the infraorbital nerve leading to a neuropraxia (Fig. 3.16). The zygomatic nerve is also frequently damaged causing anaesthesia or paraesthesia within the distribution of the zygomaticofacial and zygomaticotemporal branches. The patient may, therefore, exhibit anaesthesia of the temple, cheek, one side of the upper lip and the side of the nose. The period of anaesthesia depends on the degree of damage to the nerve, but recovery of sensation usually occurs well within six months. Symptoms suggesting damage to nerves passing through the superior orbital fissure should be regarded with caution as they may be associated with a more severe orbital injury needing careful evaluation.

Interference with mandibular excursion

When the zygomatic complex is displaced inwards, it may impinge on the coronoid process of the mandible and interfere with mandibular movements. If, as is usual, the mouth was closed at the time of injury, the patient may be unable fully to open the mouth. More rarely, if the mandible is widely open at the time of injury, the zygomatic bone may be driven in to such an extent that it is impossible for the patient to close the mouth. Lateral excursion and protrusion of the mandible to the fractured side is always impaired in these situations.

Diplopia

Diplopia is a potentially serious feature of some fractures of the zygomatic complex occurring in approximately 10% of cases. Diplopia is typically caused by interference with the action of extraocular muscles, which in most cases results from oedema and haemorrhage in and around the muscles. This type of diplopia is usually temporary, but when there has been actual damage to the extraocular muscles or to their nerve supply recovery is less certain.

Alteration of the ocular level as a result of injury may result in diplopia due to the alteration of the visual axes. Whether this occurs depends on the amount of displacement and the level at which the fracture occurs in the lateral wall of the orbit. The level of the globe is normally maintained by a condensation of the periocular connective tissue known as the suspensory ligament of Lockwood. This passes from its medial attachment on the lacrimal bone to be inserted laterally into Whitnall's tubercle situated on the inner aspect of the zygomatic bone just below the frontozygomatic suture. If the fracture passes inferior to Whitnall's tubercle, the zygomatic bone can be grossly displaced downwards without significant alteration in the level of the globe of the eye that is maintained in place by Lockwood's suspensory ligament. However, if the fracture occurs above Whitnall's tubercle and the bone is significantly displaced downwards, the globe will drop, resulting in vertical ocular dystopia (Fig. 3.19). The upper lid follows it and produces a characteristic 'hooding' of the globe or pseudoptosis, a physical sign that is exacerbated if there is enophthalmos and which becomes more obvious as the initial oedema subsides (see Fig. 3.17).

Diplopia can be tested by holding a finger or object at least an arm's length in front of the eyes and asking the patient to report double vision as the finger is moved. Diplopia recorded closer to the patient than one arm's length may not be clinically significant. It is not for example significant if reading is unaffected. Diplopia should be recorded in each of the nine positions of gaze.

A Hess chart is the most useful clinical tool for measuring the progress or otherwise of patients with double vision. The Hess chart records the range of movement of each individual eye. It shows which of the extra-ocular muscles is functioning abnormally and by repeating the examination the progress of the diplopia can be monitored. Rapid improvement indicates that double vision was caused by temporary muscle oedema. If, however, the Hess chart remains unchanged in the first week, this implies more permanent damage, a finding that will influence decisions as regards treatment.

Enophthalmos

Enophthalmos is a troublesome sequel in some fractures of the zygomatic complex. This sinking inward of the eye may itself be a cause of diplopia, although this is uncommon. Enophthalmos occurring immediately after injury is the result of an increase in the volume of the orbit due to fracture of its walls. It is made worse by herniation of fat from the orbit, usually through a defect in the floor or the thin lamina papyracea of the medial wall. Fat can also escape from the orbit via the inferior orbital fissure without there being evidence of bony injury in that area.

The anatomy of the tissues supporting the globe of the eye is quite complex. They comprise a network of connective tissue organized into fibrous septa within the orbital fat. Condensation of this connective tissue also constitutes the suspensory ligament and comprises part of the 'cone' formed by the extrinsic ocular muscles. Fibrosis of this supporting tissue can cause displacement of the globe as a contributing factor in late-developing enophthalmos.

Computed tomographic scanners can be used to measure precisely the volume of the orbit and its various soft tissue components. Comparisons between the fat volume of injured and normal orbits have demonstrated conclusively that fat atrophy is not a significant feature in most patients with early post-traumatic enophthalmos. Acute enophthalmos is caused either by escape of orbital fat or an increase in the volume of the bony orbit, or a combination of both. Fractures that involve the orbital floor often contribute to an increased orbital volume by producing a change in the sagittal contour

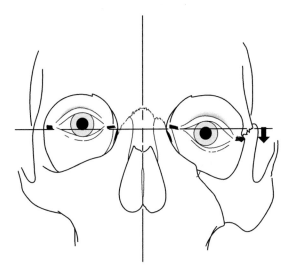

Figure 3.19 Diagram illustrating how inferior displacement of Whitnall's tubercle with the attached Lockwood's suspensory ligament leads to alteration in the level of the globe.

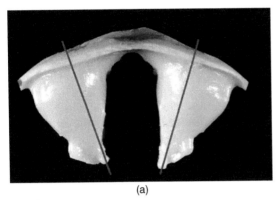

(a)

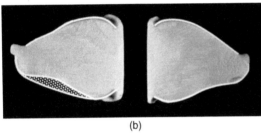

(b)

Figure 3.20 (a) Acrylic model produced from an impression of both orbital cavities viewed from above. Note that the medial walls are parallel whilst the lateral walls diverge at approximately 40–45° from the sagittal plane. (b) Oblique sagittal sections of both orbits as illustrated by red lines in (a). The normal sigmoid contour of the floor is demonstrated on the right. The typical loss of contour caused by a fracture involving the orbital floor is shown on the left. The stippled area represents the increase in orbital volume that results.

of the posterior part of the floor from a convex to a concave outline. Care needs to be taken to detect and correct this deformity if enophthalmos is to be prevented (Fig. 3.20).

Intra-oral signs

Sometimes, as the zygomatic bone is driven in, the entire maxilla is 'sprung' down without being fractured and there may be premature contact of the occlusion in the molar area on the injured side. Comminution of the outer walls of the maxillary antrum may damage the anterior, middle or posterior superior dental nerves, with resulting anaesthesia of the teeth and gums.

There is often marked ecchymosis in the upper buccal sulcus in the region of the zygomatic buttress. There is also tenderness on palpation over the zygomatic buttress area intra-orally, and sometimes crepitus may be felt. A summary of the possible clinical findings in fractures of the zygomatic complex is given in Table 3.4.

Table 3.4 Summary of clinical findings in zygomatic complex fractures.

- Flattening of cheek
- Swelling of cheek
- Anaesthesia of cheek, temple, upper teeth and gingiva
- Periorbital haematoma
- Sub-conjunctival haemorrhage
- Tenderness over orbital rim and frontozygomatic suture
- Step deformity of infraorbital margin
- Palpable separation at frontozygomatic suture
- Ecchymosis and tenderness intra-orally over zygomatic buttress
- Limitation of ocular movement
- Diplopia

Fractures of the zygomatic arch

Isolated fractures of the zygomatic arch are uncommon. They can be divided into two main varieties:
1 Triple fracture of the arch with a depressed 'V-type' of displacement.
2 Comminution of the arch.

In the V-type of displacement the apex of the V may impinge on the coronoid process and impede mandibular movements, especially lateral excursion to the injured side. In the absence of surgical correction this depression persists and constitutes a cosmetic deformity (Fig. 3.21).

When the zygomatic arch is comminuted, the fragments usually reposition themselves presumably as a result of movements of the temporalis muscle and coronoid process beneath them. Signs and symptoms may be minimal or absent.

Fractures of the zygomatic arch may coexist with fractures of the zygomatic bone. In such cases, the distinguishing features of the zygomatic arch fractures are obscured by the more gross physical signs associated with the zygomatic bone fractures.

When the zygomatic arch is fractured in isolation without fracturing the zygomatic bone at its frontozygomatic and zygomaticomaxillary suture lines the only visible evidence of fracture is a depression over the arch perhaps associated with limitation of mandibular excursion to the injured side and possible interference with mandibular opening or closing. The depression is obvious immediately after fracture of the arch, but it often becomes obscured by oedema shortly after injury only to become visible again when the swelling subsides in about a week. No other physical signs and symptoms typical of a fracture of the zygomatic bone are present.

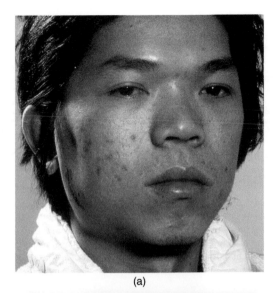

(a)

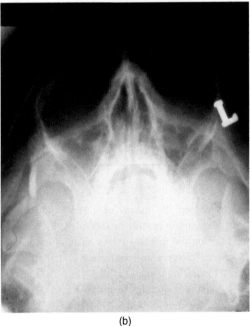

(b)

Figure 3.21 (a) Marked indentation of right cheek due to an isolated fracture of the zygomatic arch. (b) Occipitomental radiograph demonstrating the depressed 'V-type' triple fracture of the arch.

Isolated orbital floor fractures

The orbit is said to be roughly pyramidal in shape with its apex at the optic foramen, but as the junctions between its walls are rounded it does in fact more resemble a cone. It is described as having a medial and lateral wall, a roof and a floor. The medial wall is very thin and beneath it lie the ethmoidal air cells. Both the lateral wall and the roof are relatively thick, but the floor of the orbit that slopes upwards towards the optic foramen is also extremely thin, particularly in the region of the infraorbital groove that anteriorly becomes the infraorbital canal (see Fig. 3.15).

The orbital floor is made up of the orbital portion of the maxillary bone and part of the zygomatic bone. It is bounded laterally by the inferior orbital fissure. Posteriorly, it is made up of the orbital process of the palatine bone and a small portion of the ethmoid bone. Medially the floor is bounded by the lacrimal bone.

The eyeball normally protrudes slightly beyond the orbital rim and it is suspended by Lockwood's ligament. The eyeball itself is relatively tough and is filled with incompressible vitreous humour. Apart from the extra-ocular muscles the remainder of the orbital cavity is largely filled with fat.

When an object of slightly greater diameter than the orbital rim strikes the protruding incompressible eyeball, the rapid increase in intra-orbital pressure results in fracture of the weak part of the orbital floor. This type of injury is commonly called an 'orbital blow-out fracture'. However, this type of 'blow-out' can also be caused experimentally in the cadaver by a sharp blow to the infraorbital rim. Rarely a 'blow-in' fracture, (inward buckling of the orbital floor) can occur. This is usually seen in children, also resulting from trauma to the inferior orbital rim. It is therefore preferable to refer to all these injuries as 'isolated' orbital floor fractures and to remember that the history of the injury is important in diagnosis.

In fractures caused by the blow-out mechanisms, the fragments of bone are displaced downwards into the antral cavity remaining attached to the orbital periosteum rather like a trap-door. The periorbital fat tends to herniate through the defect and this has the effect of interfering with the action of the inferior rectus and inferior oblique muscles that are contained within the same fascial sheath. This tethering effect is amplified by the fibrous septa present within the orbital fat. If a large enough amount of orbital fat is displaced through the orbital floor defect it may result in enophthalmos.

It should be remembered that the increased hydraulic pressure transmitted by the orbital contents can also cause rupture of the medial wall of the orbit with displacement of fat in this direction. Orbital contents may also herniate through the inferior orbital fissure by a similar mechanism, and both of these injuries will contribute to immediate or residual enophthalmos.

As has been mentioned, the actions of the inferior oblique and inferior rectus muscles may be impeded in the longer term by tethering following fibrous tissue formation. Interference with the action of these muscles prevents upward movement and outward rotation of the eye with resulting double vision in these directions of gaze.

Signs and symptoms

The key feature of the isolated orbital floor fracture is the absence of obvious bony damage to the zygomatic bone and arch even though clinical examination suggests such an injury might have occurred. In the immediate post-traumatic phase the characteristic signs and symptoms are masked by oedema and ecchymosis, both within and around the orbit. There is circumorbital and subconjunctival ecchymosis that may be associated with surgical emphysema caused by leakage of air from the paranasal air sinuses. If the lamina papyracea of the ethmoid bone is ruptured surgical emphysema may result from the patient blowing their nose violently. In the acute phase the eye may be proptosed and there is frequently paraesthesia within the distribution of the infraorbital nerve.

Owing to the generalized oedema diplopia may initially be present in all directions of gaze but as the swelling settles it remains present only on looking upwards. If there has been a large herniation of orbital contents through the floor of the orbit clinical enophthalmos may be apparent or it may be demonstrated by observing retraction of the globe of the eye on attempted upward gaze. The tethering of the inferior muscles can be further demonstrated by the forced duction test, which may be carried out under local or general anaesthesia (Fig. 3.22). Fine toothed dissecting forceps are inserted under the globe of the eye via the inferior conjunctival fornix and the insertion of the inferior rectus is gently grasped enabling the globe to be forcibly rotated upwards and its freedom of movement compared with the opposite side. Any increased resistance is readily appreciated and is diagnostic of muscle tethering.

In these circumstances vertical diplopia will be present, which will be maximal on extreme upward gaze. It is essential to measure this interference with

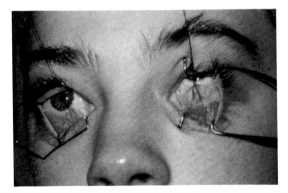

Figure 3.22 Forced duction test under general anaesthesia in a young patient with an isolated ('blow-out') fracture of the right orbital floor. A traction suture has been passed round the insertion of each inferior rectus muscle. The lack of passive upward movement of the right eye due to tethering is clearly seen.

Table 3.5 Summary of possible clinical findings in isolated orbital floor fractures.

- Periorbital ecchymosis
- Sub-conjunctival haemorrhage
- Diplopia
- Limitation of eye movement especially in upward gaze
- Globe retraction on upward gaze
- Enophthalmos
- Surgical emphysema of eyelids
- Paraesthesia within distribution of infraorbital nerve

orbital movement by means of a Hess chart and to monitor any improvement, or lack of it, by repeating the test during the first 7–10 days after injury. Isolated orbital floor fractures are confirmed and their extent delineated by CT imaging.

The key clinical findings in isolated fractures of the orbital floor are summarized in Table 3.5.

Fractures of the nose and naso-orbito-ethmoid complex

The bony and cartilaginous skeleton of the nose is often referred to as the nasal 'pyramid'. The nasal bones are relatively thick superiorly where they are attached to the frontal bone, but are thinner inferiorly where the upper lateral cartilages are attached. Hence they are more susceptible to fractures lower down.

The upper lateral cartilages are attached to the undersurface of the nasal bones. This is a key area in both aesthetics and function. Injuries in this region can result in collapse of the bones and/or upper lateral cartilages, which is not only cosmetically disfiguring but can impair nasal breathing. The upper lateral cartilages articulate with the lower lateral (or alar) cartilages. This overall arrangement is sometimes referred to as the 'nasal valve'. The paired lower lateral cartilages along with the septum define the position and shape of the nasal tip. The septum is a key structure in maintaining nasal projection and the midline position of the nose.

With low energy impacts the nasal bones often fracture in isolation, but with higher energy injuries it is more usual for fractures to extend and involve the frontal process of the maxilla and the lower part of the medial wall of the orbit. In the latter case, there may be comminution of the lacrimal bones and the orbital plate of the ethmoid with associated lateral displacement of the medial canthus of the eye.

Nasal complex fractures can be divided into three planes of injury depending on the force applied (Fig. 3.23). In simple terms the first plane involves the nasal tip only, the second plane involves the whole of the external nose anterior to the orbital rim, while the third plane is a much more severe injury involving the medial orbital wall and sometimes the anterior cranial fossa. These latter injuries are now distinguished as fractures of the naso-orbito-ethmoid complex. Such a fracture causes considerable depression of the central part of the face without any disturbance of the occlusion.

Fractures of the nasal region usually involve the nasal septum. Sometimes the septal cartilage is merely dislodged from its groove in the vomer but frequently the cartilaginous septum is fractured in a C-shaped pattern. In more serious injuries the cartilage may be comminuted and the vomer and perpendicular plates of the ethmoid may be fractured. In very severe injuries there may be cerebrospinal fluid rhinorrhoea.

The displacement of the nose depends on the direction of the fracturing force. Force applied laterally to the nose leads to the nasal bones and associated portions of the frontal processes of the maxillae being displaced to one side. At the same time, the septal cartilage that is attached to the inner aspect of the nasal bones is subjected to a strain, which causes it to fracture or be detached from its groove in the vomer. Force applied anteriorly over the bridge of the nose

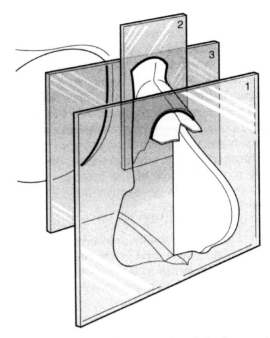

Figure 3.23 Diagrammatic representation of the three possible planes of nasal fracture. 1. Nasal tip only. 2. Nasal bones. 3. Naso-orbito-ethmoid complex. (Adapted from Stranc 1979. Reproduced with permission of L&W)

leads to the nasal bones being driven inwards, while the frontal processes of the maxillae and lacrimal bones fracture and are splayed outwards. The attachments of the medial canthal ligaments of the eye are displaced laterally producing traumatic telecanthus, the severity of which relates directly to the degree of impaction. All of this results in a flattened, depressed nose, and again the underlying septal cartilage and the vomer and perpendicular and cribriform plates of the ethmoid may be variously involved.

If untreated, the lateral type of injury will result in a deviation of the nose to one side, with chronic airway obstruction. Untreated anterior-type injuries leave a flattened nose with thickened bridge. More severe injuries leave the patient with telecanthus, chronic airway obstruction and often disturbance of lacrimal drainage (Fig. 3.24).

Signs and symptoms of fractures of the nasal complex

In the recent injury there is invariably epistaxis, and when the blood has clotted there may be a discharge of clear serum. If the cribriform plate of the ethmoid has

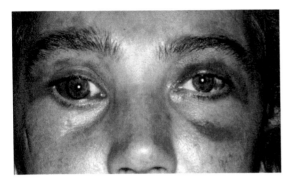

Figure 3.24 Fracture of nasal bones and inter-orbital region following frontal impact (plane No. 3 in Fig. 3.23). Note broadening and flattening of nasal bridge with inferior displacement of right inner canthus.

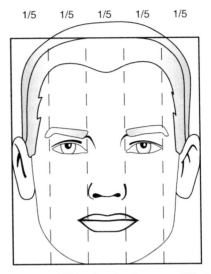

Figure 3.25 'Rule of fifths' showing the assumed ideal proportions of the face on frontal view. This may be of use in assessing traumatic telecanthus and naso-orbito-ethmoid deformity once swelling has resolved.

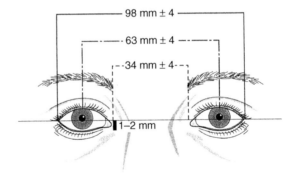

Figure 3.26 Normal intercanthal and interpupillary measurements (Caucasian).

been comminuted, there may be a cerebrospinal fluid leak. The tissue over the bridge of the nose is thin and the fragments of nasal bone may penetrate the skin, rendering the fracture compound. If the nostrils are gently cleared of blood a nasal speculum can be used to inspect the nasal septum that may be visibly torn or displaced, or there may be a septal haematoma. Much of the skeletal displacement may be masked by the overlying oedema.

It is usual for there to be bilateral circumorbital ecchymosis and possibly subconjunctival haemorrhage, more marked on the medial aspect. The entire nose may be seen to be deviated to one side following a lateral injury while an anterior fracturing force produces a saddle-type depression of the bridge.

Previous untreated fractures can result in a difficult diagnostic problem, particularly when the patient is unable to give a lucid history. Palpation of the nasal skeleton will usually distinguish a fresh injury from a previous deformity. The underlying nasal bones will be mobile and sometimes comminuted. Sharp step deformities may be felt and the bony complex will be acutely tender. When there is extensive comminution, the entire area gives the feeling 'lead shot' under the palpating finger.

It is important to determine whether the medial canthal ligament of the eye is displaced, as it may be in those fractures that involve the deeper bony components of the medial orbital wall. As an approximate assessment a 'rule of fifths' can be used, although its usefulness may be limited if there is significant facial swelling (Fig. 3.25). It is better to make a formal measurement of the intercanthal distances and also the distance of each medial canthus from the midline, as the displacement may be unilateral. Generally speaking, an inner intercanthal measurement greater than 35 mm is indicative of canthal displacement (Fig. 3.26).

Pre-injury photographs may be extremely useful in some cases, especially if a pre-existing deformity is suspected. A summary of the possible clinical findings in fractures of the nasal bones and naso-orbito-ethmoid complex is outlined in Table 3.6.

Table 3.6 Summary of possible clinical findings in nasal complex fractures.

- Bruising of skin over nasal bones
- Laceration of skin of bridge of nose
- Bilateral medial orbital ecchymosis
- Epistaxis
- Deformity of nose and inter-orbital area
- Crepitus of bones of nasal complex
- Unilateral or bilateral telecanthus
- Airway obstruction
- Septal deviation
- Septal laceration or haematoma
- Cerebrospinal rhinorrhoea

Central midface fractures involving the dentoalveolar component (Le Fort type fractures)

Low-level fractures (Le Fort I)

Low-level fractures of the midface are more precisely defined by the Le Fort classification than the more complex fractures at a higher level. The fracture may occur as a single entity or in association with other fractures of the midface. It is not infrequently present in association with a downward displaced fracture of the zygomatic complex. In this situation the upper tooth-bearing segment is either wholly or partially sprung downwards and the fracture may easily be missed by the unaware. A Le Fort I fracture that often escapes diagnosis is the impacted type, which results from violence transmitted via a blow to the lower jaw and is often therefore associated with a fracture of the mandible.

Signs and symptoms

In a recent injury there may be slight swelling of the upper lip, but there is none of the massive oedema of the face that characterizes Le Fort II and III type fractures. Typically ecchymosis is present in the buccal sulcus beneath each zygomatic arch. The occlusion is disturbed and a variable amount of mobility may be found in the tooth-bearing segment of the maxilla. Some low level fractures are so mobile that the whole fragment drops and the patient may have to keep the mouth slightly open to accommodate the increased vertical dimension of the bite. This situation may result from a direct blow from a sharp object in the front of

the mouth above the apices of the teeth. When this happens a soft-tissue laceration is often present, and in extreme cases the resulting down fracture of the maxilla may be so gross that it may be possible to see directly into the nares and the maxillary antra through the upper lip.

Most low level fractures are not as mobile as this. Indeed the impacted type of fracture may be almost immobile and it is only by grasping the maxillary teeth and applying slight but firm movement, that a characteristic grate can be felt that is diagnostic of the fracture (Fig. 3.27). An attempt to move the maxillary cheek teeth apart should be made in the same way to make sure there is no associated split in the palate. This usually occurs, but not always, in the line of the median palatal suture and typically results from a force transmitted upwards via the mandibular teeth. If this is present midline bruising of the palate may be evident or even a split of the mucosa (Fig. 3.28).

In the impacted type of fracture there may be damage to the cusps of individual teeth, usually in the premolar region, caused by the impaction of the mandibular teeth against them. Percussion of the upper teeth results in a distinctive 'cracked-pot' sound, similar to that produced when cracked china is tapped with a spoon. This sign is present whenever there is a fracture of the central middle third of the face, but is particularly valuable in the diagnosis of Le Fort I fractures. Table 3.7 lists the possible clinical findings in low level Le Fort I fractures.

All possible variations of open and closed type fractures may occur and it is possible to see the condition unilaterally when it involves only one maxilla, the tooth-bearing portion being split along the median palatal suture. The complete Le Fort I fracture is often associated with a split in the palate sometimes along more than one line so that each of two or more fragments may be mobile. Multiple alveolar fractures of this nature are frequently complicated by damaged or subluxed teeth.

High level fractures (Le Fort II and III type)

As mentioned previously distinguishing between these fracture patterns by clinical examination is of little practical value in determining treatment. The precise pattern of the bony injury is better defined by appropriate CT imaging than by clinical examination. The signs and symptoms are so similar that they can be considered together. The two types of fracture frequently coexist,

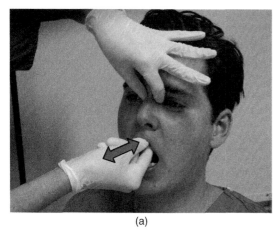

(a)

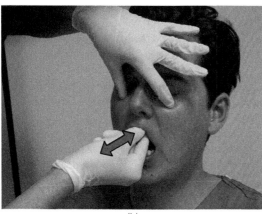

(b)

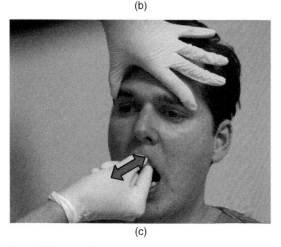

(c)

Figure 3.27 Testing for maxillary mobility by grasping the anterior alveolus, or placing fingers in the palatal vault, and 'rocking' the maxilla (a–c). Lack of simultaneous palpable mobility at the nasal bridge denotes a low level maxillary fracture (Le Fort I) whilst coexistent mobility at the infra-orbital rims or nasal bridge denotes a high level monobloc fracture (Le Fort II or III type).

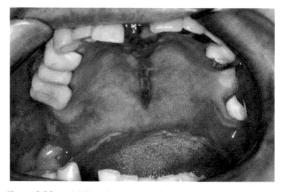

Figure 3.28 Mid-line laceration of the palatal mucosa in a patient with a split Le Fort I type fracture. The traumatic diastema between the central incisor teeth is also obvious.

Table 3.7 Summary of possible clinical findings in Le Fort I fractures.

- Mobility of whole of dentoalveolar segment of upper jaw
- Palpable crepitation in upper buccal sulcus
- 'Cracked pot' percussion note from upper teeth
- Haematoma intra-orally over root of zygoma
- Ecchymosis or laceration in palate
- Fractured cusps of cheek teeth
- Bruising of upper lip and lower half of midface

one with the other, or with associated Le Fort I or zygomatic complex fractures.

Signs and symptoms common to Le Fort II and III fractures

Classically these fractures are associated with gross oedema of the soft tissues overlying the middle third of the facial skeleton, giving rise to the characteristic 'moon-face' appearance. This 'ballooning' of the features is not seen in isolated Le Fort I fractures, and occurs within a very short time of injury (Fig. 3.29).

Bilateral circumorbital ecchymosis is invariably a feature of both fractures and this also develops quite rapidly after injury. The associated rapid swelling of the eyelids makes examination of the eyes difficult but it is absolutely essential to do this at an early stage to exclude damage to the globe of the eye. Steady but gentle pressure upon the swollen eyelids, sustained for 1 or 2 minutes, will displace the oedema sufficiently to allow them to be parted. This manoeuvre also allows the orbital rim to be palpated with accuracy.

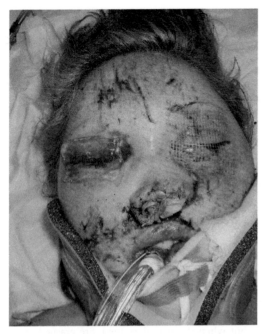

Figure 3.29 Intubated patient with multiple midface fractures showing the gross facial oedema and bilateral circumorbital ecchymosis typically seen soon after this type of injury.

Subconjunctival ecchymosis usually develops rapidly, but it sometimes requires several hours to become fully established. Subconjunctival haemorrhage tends to occur adjacent to those parts of the orbit where fracture has occurred, but the pattern is so variable that it is of little diagnostic value

Oedema of the conjunctiva, known as chemosis, is frequently seen in association with a periorbital haematoma. This causes the swollen conjunctiva to bulge out from between the eyelids, a feature that becomes more obvious as the eyelid swelling subsides.

Both Le Fort II and III type fractures involve the orbit and if they coexist, the orbit itself is usually extensively damaged. It is essential that the eyes are examined at an early stage by an ophthalmologist. Fortunately, it is extremely rare for the fracturing force to damage the optic nerve, as the nerve is protected by a strong ring of compact bone that forms the apical foramen and the fracture line goes around the foramen rather than through it. Nevertheless vision can be impaired as a result of the injury, and it is therefore imperative to test it as soon as possible. Careful note should be made of any variation in the size of the pupils, which may be the

result of peripheral damage to the oculomotor nerve in the superior orbital fissure, or more seriously may be an early sign of intracranial haemorrhage.

In the early stage of the injury it is often difficult to test ocular movements or test for diplopia, but diplopia is usually present and ocular movements may be limited.

Both fracture types pass through the nasal complex of bones at their base, and may extend backwards to involve the cribriform plate area. The nasal complex itself exhibits varying degrees of comminution, but in general when a Le Fort III type fracture is present, the damage in this region tends to be more extensive than in the Le Fort II fracture alone. Usually the pattern of nasal fracture is characteristic of an anterior rather than a lateral blow with flattening of the bridge and spreading of the intercanthal distance.

The nares tend to be filled with clotted blood and there may be a steady trickle of straw-coloured fluid from the nose, suggesting a cerebrospinal fluid leak mixed with serum (see Fig 3.13).

In both types of fracture, the bones of the middle third of the face have been separated from the inclined plane of the base of the skull and forced downwards and backwards to a variable degree. A very large impacting force tends to cause comminution of the bones in the anterior parts of the face, rather than an increase in the posterior displacement, a fact demonstrated quite clearly by Le Fort in his original experiments. The backward and downward displacement of the tuberosity area of the maxilla and palate is therefore rarely, if ever, sufficient to obstruct the nasopharynx as often described. However, even slight downward displacement of the maxillary molar teeth is sufficient to cause gagging of the occlusion, and there will usually be some retroposition of the maxilla as a whole.

Occasionally there is wide separation of the middle third of the face from the skull base. Clinicians frequently refer to a 'floating' maxilla in such cases. When this occurs, there is usually an additional fracture at the Le Fort I level, although the maxillae may be very loose in some pure Le Fort II and III type fractures. In such cases there will be extreme lengthening of the face (see Fig.3.30). It should be appreciated that extreme mobility of Le Fort II and III fractures is the exception rather than the rule. A lesser degree of mobility of the middle face is readily detected by grasping the anterior maxillary alveolus and gently moving it forwards and

Table 3.8 Summary of possible clinical findings common to Le Fort II and III fractures.

- Gross oedema of soft tissues over the middle third of the facial skeleton
- Bilateral circum-orbital ecchymosis
- Bilateral sub-conjunctival haemorrhage
- Nasal deformity
- Bleeding from nose or nasal obstruction from clotted blood
- Cerebrospinal fluid rhinorrhoea sometimes appreciated by the patient as a salty taste
- 'Dish-face' deformity of the face with occasional noticeable lengthening
- Limitation of ocular movement with possible diplopia and enophthalmos
- Retropositioning of maxillae, so that anterior teeth do not meet, and there is gagging on the posterior teeth
- Difficulty in opening mouth, and sometimes inability to move the lower jaw
- Mobility of the upper jaw
- Occasional haematoma of palate. Blood clot frequently present in palatal vault
- 'Cracked-pot' sound on tapping teeth

Table 3.9 Summary of possible clinical findings peculiar Le Fort II type fractures.

- Step deformity at infraorbital margins
- Mobility of midface detectable at nasal bridge and infraorbital margins
- Anaesthesia or paraesthesia of cheek
- Possible diplopia
- Pupils tend to be level unless there is gross unilateral enophthalmos
- Nasal bones move with midface as a whole but often otherwise intact
- Cerebrospinal fluid rhinorrhoea may not be clinically detectable
- No tenderness over, or disorganization and mobility of zygomatic bones and arch

backwards. Tapping of the upper teeth will give the characteristic 'cracked-pot' sound.

In both Le Fort II and III type fractures there may be extensive bruising of the soft palate, particularly when the maxillae have separated in the midline. Blood clot frequently accumulates around the teeth and particularly in the vault of the palate, where it causes the patient considerable discomfort.

A summary of the clinical findings common to both Le Fort II and III fractures is given in Table 3.8.

Signs and symptoms peculiar to Le Fort II fractures

The most obvious difference between Le Fort II and III fractures, from the clinical point of view, is the detection of a step deformity in the bone of the infraorbital margin. This is made more apparent when the zygomatic complex on each side is intact.

As the fracture line passes across the inferior orbital rim, there is likely to be associated injury to the infraorbital nerve resulting in anaesthesia or paraesthesia of the cheek. Similarly the fracture line in the orbital floor may result in limitation of orbital movement in an upward direction with diplopia and possibly enophthalmos.

Because the line of fracture is below the lateral attachment of the suspensory ligament of Lockwood,

alteration of the pupil level does not occur unless there is an associated fracture of the zygomatic complex.

Gagging of the occlusion and retropositioning of the maxilla as a whole will be noted on intra-oral examination, but when the maxillary teeth are grasped, it will be noted that the midfacial skeleton moves as a pyramid, the movement being detected by palpation at the infraorbital margins and nasal bridge.

The Le Fort II fracture may be impacted in the same manner as the Le Fort I, in which case little or no mobility can be detected. There is frequently a midline or paramedian split in the pyramidal block.

The passage of the fracture line across the zygomatic buttress gives rise to haematoma formation in the upper buccal sulcus on each side, adjacent to the first and second molar teeth. Unless the fracturing force was applied directly to the nasal region, the comminution of this part of the pyramidal block is usually minimal. There is less danger of fracture of the anterior cranial fossa and cerebrospinal fluid rhinorrhoea is therefore not a constant clinical finding. However, when a Le Fort II type fracture is present, it must be assumed that a breach of the dura mater has occurred, even if overt leakage of cerebrospinal fluid is not detected.

A summary of the clinical findings peculiar to Le Fort II fractures is given in Table 3.9.

Signs and symptoms peculiar to Le Fort III fractures

Superficially the Le Fort III type fracture appears very similar to the Le Fort II fracture, but it is usually obvious that the injury is very much more severe. It is, however, very unusual to find a Le Fort III fracture occurring in isolation. A frontal blow of sufficient force to separate the facial bones at the Le Fort III level usually produces coexistent fracture at Le Fort II and I levels, together with extensive comminution of the nasal complex. Indeed in injuries of this severity the Le Fort classification becomes meaningless other than as a general guide to the fracture pattern. An uncommon isolated Le Fort III fracture is most likely to be produced by an oblique blow from a lateral direction in which case there may be tilting and some lengthening of the facial skeleton due to separation at the frontozygomatic suture line.

The clinical features of the Le Fort III fracture are superficially similar to the Le Fort II pattern, but there are clear differences as described next.

There is tenderness and often separation at the frontozygomatic sutures. The amount of separation may not be symmetrical in which case the facial skeleton will be tilted to the side opposite to the direction of the fracturing force. Separation of both fronto-zygomatic sutures produces lengthening of the face and lowering of the ocular level, due to the fracture passing above Whitnall's tubercle. As one or both eyes drop, the upper lid follows the globe down, producing unilateral or bilateral pseudoptosis described as 'hooding' of the eyes (Fig. 3.30).

A complete fracture at the Le Fort III level cannot occur without fracture of each zygomatic arch and coincident independent fracture of one or other zygomatic complex almost invariably occurs. The displacement of the zygomatic complex will be detectable by palpation, which will reveal flattening and a step deformity at the infraorbital margin. In addition, if a finger and thumb are placed over the frontonasal suture region and the dentoalveolar portion of the upper jaw grasped with the other hand, movement of the entire face can be demonstrated. As mentioned previously the zygomatic bones may often be independently mobile.

Intra-orally there is gagging of the occlusion in the molar area, as in other fractures of the middle third. When lateral displacement has taken place, the molar teeth will be found to be gagged on one side only with a posterior open bite on the opposite side and deviation of the upper midline. The entire occlusal plane may have dropped, holding the mandible open, a dramatic but rather unusual finding.

A very loose Le Fort III fracture is usually associated with disruption of the cribriform plate area, and this type of fracture may therefore produce a profuse cerebrospinal fluid rhinorrhoea. In this situation

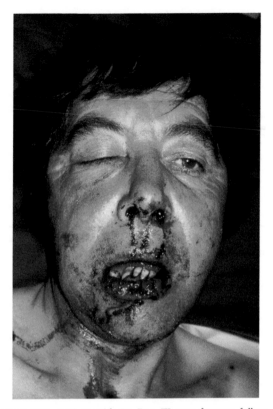

Figure 3.30 Patient with Le Fort III type fracture following a lateral blow to the midface. There is separation of the fronto-zygomatic sutures, lengthening of the face and deviation of the naso-maxillary complex to the left. The ocular level on the right has fallen with the upper lid following it to produce a pseudoptosis known as 'hooding'.

the possibility of an intracranial aerocele must be considered.

A summary of the clinical findings peculiar to Le Fort II fractures is given in Table 3.10.

Unilateral and complex midfacial fractures

It is possible for a unilateral fracture of the middle third of the facial skeleton to occur, which may be of the Le Fort I, II or III variety. In this situation the physical signs are similar to those already described but they are of course, only present on one side.

The description of the clinical signs and symptoms shows the complexity of much midfacial trauma, particularly after high energy impacts. Many combinations of fracture patterns may be present that make the standard Le Fort classification of fractures lines of limited value.

Table 3.10 Summary of possible clinical findings peculiar to Le Fort III fractures*.

- Step deformity at infraorbital margins
- Mobility of midface detectable at nasal bridge *and* infraorbital margins
- Anaesthesia or paraesthesia of cheek
- Possible diplopia
- Pupils tend to be level unless there is gross unilateral enophthalmos
- Nasal bones move with midface as a whole but often otherwise intact
- Cerebrospinal fluid rhinorrhoea may not be clinically detectable
- No tenderness or disorganization and mobility of zygomatic bones and arch

*Note: Le Fort III fractures, as classically described, rarely present clinically as 'monobloc' fractures

Complex midfacial fractures are most readily evaluated by modern CT imaging and this is essential for accurate treatment planning. Once it has been established clinically that there is multiple fracturing of the midfacial skeleton there is little to be gained by attempting to determine the exact fracture pattern from a clinical examination alone.

Further reading

Fehrenbach MJ, Herring SW, Thomas P. *Illustrated Anatomy of the Head and Neck.* 4th Edn. ISBN 978–1-4377–2419–6 Publisher: WB Saunders, 2012.

Le Fort R. Experimental study of fractures of the upper jaw. *Plast Reconstr Surg.* 1972:50(5):497–506 and 1972:50(6)600–607. (English translations by P. Tessier of the original French papers published by René Le Fort in Revue de Chirurgie in 1901.)

Perry M, Holmes S. *Atlas of Operative Maxillofacial Trauma Surgery.* ISBN 9978-1-4471-2855-7. Springer, 2014

Romanes GJ. *Cunningham's Manual of Practical Anatomy: Volume 3. Head and Neck and Brain.* ISBN 0192631403. Oxford University Press, Nov. 1986.

Ward-Booth P, Hausaman J-E, and Schendel S. *Maxillofacial Surgery* (two-volume set). ISBN 0443058539. Churchill Livingstone, Oct. 2006.

Ward-Booth P, Eppley B, Schmelzheisen R. *Maxillofacial Trauma and Esthetic Reconstruction.* 2nd Edn. ISBN 1437724205. Saunders. Nov. 2011.

CHAPTER 4

Imaging

The management of many facial fractures has improved considerably as a result of advances in imaging techniques, in particular the increased availability and refinement of computed tomographic (CT) scanning and magnetic resonance imaging (MRI). Although these modalities are widely available in economically well-developed countries it should be remembered that there are still many fewer advantaged countries where major maxillofacial trauma is common and where most hospitals will still have to rely largely on traditional radiographic imaging. Indeed plain radiographs supply good diagnostic information in the majority of fractures and they still provide the foundation of imaging. In many patients they may be sufficient on their own, and in others they can provide an indication for the supplementary use of other modalities such as CT and MRI. Generally speaking most injuries due to low energy impacts will not require CT scanning as routine, but very few patients will be managed without resort to plain radiographs.

Imaging in the initial management of the trauma patient

All clinicians who treat facial fractures will be familiar with the scenario of a patient transferred to their care having already had a large number of radiographs taken; often inappropriately prescribed, of poor quality and of little or no diagnostic value. It is therefore important that all doctors working in accident departments understand some basic principles when it comes to requesting radiographs of facial injuries. Apart from the obvious cost savings, a rational informed approach will also prevent seriously injured patients from being subjected to prolonged and unnecessary imaging to the possible detriment of their overall care.

Clinically stable patients

The majority of patients with facial bone fractures have injuries confined to the face and are usually ambulatory or clinically stable. In this situation extensive radiographic examination in a busy accident department is unnecessary and usually relatively non-productive. Prioritizing is important, particularly in patients with multiple injuries, and most patients with facial injuries do not need immediate imaging. If a facial fracture is clinically obvious, for instance a depressed zygoma or a fractured mandible with occlusal disturbance, it is usually more important to arrange timely specialist referral than to take radiographs. If radiographs are thought necessary in the accident department, perhaps to identify or exclude a suspected fracture, then a panoral tomogram (OPT) together with a good quality occipitomental (OM) view will be sufficient to diagnose the presence of most common facial fractures. If these views show an obvious or suspected fracture a more comprehensive radiographic examination can be postponed until the patient is under the care of a specialist department.

Multiply injured patients

With the widespread adoption of Advanced Trauma Life Support (ATLS American College of Surgeons) and other trauma protocols it is now routine for a multiply injured patient to undergo a series of standard investigations on admission. These will usually include various plain radiographs as listed in Table 4.1.

Skull radiographs may still be requested in some accident departments for patients with evidence of a closed head injury. However, there is no evidence that these plain views alter the management of the patient and modern guidelines have moved away from this as standard. Whenever a skull fracture or intracranial injury is suspected, CT is now more appropriate.

Fractures of the Facial Skeleton, Second Edition. Michael Perry, Andrew Brown and Peter Banks.
© 2015 John Wiley & Sons, Ltd. Published 2015 by John Wiley & Sons, Ltd.

Table 4.1 Commonly requested radiographs in the assessment of the multiply injured patient.

• Chest X-ray • Pelvic X-ray • Cervical spine views	sometimes collectively referred to as a 'trauma series'

Depending on local protocols other screening views may include:

• Thoracolumbar views
• Skull radiographs

CT scanning of head and torso may form part of the protocol in the management of a multiply injured patient. Every effort should be made to incorporate facial imaging into such protocols. In particular, if a patient requires CT of their head and cervical spine, and facial fractures are obvious or suspected, they should have imaging of the face at the same time (see discussion on CT in the next section).

Imaging modalities

The different modalities available for the diagnosis of facial bone fractures are discussed next before considering the specific imaging required for each possible fracture site.

Plain radiographs

It has been mentioned previously that the occipitomental projection is one of the most useful 'screening' views of the facial bones. Unfortunately in supine patients this view, along with the posterior-anterior (PA) view of the face, is often taken in the reverse direction with the tube positioned in front of the face and the film or digital sensor at the back of the head. Such views are of little use in definitive diagnosis. All posterior-anterior projections are of much better diagnostic value when taken as the name suggests, with the patient sitting upright with the film or sensor in contact with the front of the face. However, depending on their general status and other injuries, this may not be possible in all patients. Several views require the neck to be extended and therefore they cannot be taken until the patient is 'cleared' of any cervical spine injury.

Ideally, occipitomental views should be taken with the patient upright with the nose and chin in contact with the plate. Two views are usually indicated with the central beam angled at 10° and 30° above the horizontal. This throws the shadow of the dense petrous temporal bone below the projection of the maxillary sinuses. If CT scan facilities are unavailable, a Waters view may help evaluate a suspected isolated orbital floor fracture. This may be regarded as an 'incorrectly aligned' occipitomental projection. The central beam passes along the line of the orbital floor and in this case the shadow of the dense petrous temporal bone will overlap the lower aspect of the maxillary sinuses.

Other plain views that may be helpful in diagnosis and treatment planning include a lateral projection of the facial bones, a rotated PA projection and the all too often neglected occlusal and periapical dental radiographs.

It should be noted that there are a number of traditional views that are still occasionally requested even though they are of limited diagnostic value. These include the submento-vertex and reverse Townes projections. It is generally accepted that simple nasal fractures do not require radiographs at all.

Rotational and linear tomography

Tomograms are radiographs generated from machines that allow the X-ray film (or sensor) and the tube to move around the patient. The desired plane at the axis of rotation is kept in focus while the remainder of the image is blurred. Rotational panoral tomography (Orthopantomogram or OPT) is almost universally available and is routinely used in suspected fractures of the mandible. Tomograms taken with a conventional OPT machine require a cooperative patient who can stand or sit still whilst the exposure takes place, a requirement that may not be possible if they are intoxicated or have multiple injuries. Plain oblique views of the mandible can often be obtained as an alternative but it is preferable, if at all possible, to withhold definitive radiographic examination until the patient is in a better condition.

Previously traditional indications for linear tomograms of the facial region, such as suspected damage to the orbital walls or complex injuries to the temporomandibular articulation, have now largely been superseded by CT.

Computed tomography (CT)

CT scanning is now the investigation of choice in the assessment of nearly all significant trauma, especially craniofacial injuries. Most severely or multiply injured patients will probably require a CT in the early stages of their overall assessment and this should include the facial bones if obvious facial injuries are present. CT technology has rapidly evolved, not only significantly reducing radiation dosages but also reducing the acquisition times, such that imaging of the face is now quite possible as an additional procedure during the assessment of serious head or torso injuries. With newer high speed machines the short extra time required to image the face obviates previous arguments that facial CT would delay intervention in sick patients. If a patient is stable enough to undergo CT of the head or torso, they are likely to be stable enough to undergo CT of the face at the same time as well. This often avoids additional later transfers of the patient and facilitates comprehensive and coordinated treatment planning. Injuries affecting the skull base, orbital apex and ocular region in particular need rapid identification and CT is particularly useful in assessment of these areas (Table 4.2). Both axial and coronal views are indicated.

Although CT scanners are now widely available, it should be remembered that the majority of simple facial bone fractures can be diagnosed from a thorough clinical examination in conjunction with conventional radiographs. The main indications for CT of the facial skeleton in maxillofacial trauma are given in Table 4.3.

The increasing use of cone-beam computed tomography (CBCT) in dentistry has resulted in its promotion as a useful alternative to conventional CT in facial trauma, with the claim that it provides good quality images with less radiation. This may be true for some dentoalveolar injuries and mandibular fractures, although for most fractures at this level plain views are usually more than adequate. For higher level fractures conventional CT remains the investigation of choice because of superior images and greater versatility.

Table 4.2 CT scanning of the head, face and neck: possible occult injuries to be excluded.

- Cervical spine and intracranial injuries
- Anterior cranial fossa fractures/intracranial air (risk of CSF leaks)
- Complex fractures of the frontal sinus (risk of meningitis/mucocoele)
- Middle cranial fossa fractures around vascular foramina (risk of carotid dissection/ aneurysm)
- Globe rupture/vitreous haemorrhage/foreign body
- Orbital apex fractures/optic nerve compression

Table 4.3 Main indications for CT in maxillofacial trauma.

- Suspected or obvious fracture of the frontal bone.
- Extensive fractures of the midface (including naso-orbito-ethmoid and comminuted zygomatic complex fractures).
- Isolated orbital trauma.
- Displaced condylar neck fractures and complex injuries to the temporomandibular joint.
- Comminuted fractures of the mandible requiring complex repair.
- Suspected pathological fracture of the mandible.

Viewing CT scans

CT scan data can be viewed on most personal computers using appropriate software, although high resolution monitor screens are needed for the best diagnostic images. Dedicated facial scans are essential to get the maximum benefit with 'slices' of no more than 1 mm in thickness, and preferably 0.5 mm in critical areas such as the naso-orbital region. They should be assessed in all three planes. Axial (horizontal) views are especially important to assess the zygomatic arch, nasal septum, orbital apex, and medial and lateral orbital walls. Coronal views are needed to assess the orbital floor, medial orbital wall and skull base. Sagittal views are useful for assessing the posterior extent of orbital floor fractures and the skull base. Other areas of the facial skeleton can be visualized by combinations of these three views.

The computerized data can be manipulated by appropriate software to generate a three dimensional screen image that can then be rotated and viewed from various aspects to give a picture of the overall fracture configuration that may be easier for the non-radiologist to interpret (Fig. 4.1). Dimensionally accurate models can also be fabricated from this data if required and custom made implants or pre-bent fixation plates produced. However, some fine detail is usually lost in the reformatting process and conventional CT 'slices' are still required for detailed radiological assessment.

Magnetic resonance imaging (MRI)

MRI has little if any application in the diagnosis of acute facial trauma. However, it can be helpful in the evaluation of cerebrospinal fluid leaks, suspected intracranial injuries and spinal injuries. It may also be indicated for assessing the orbital contents and for functional intra-articular imaging in temporomandibular joint injuries.

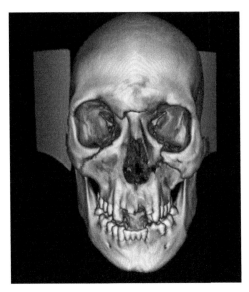

Figure 4.1 Reformatted three-dimensional image generated from CT scans showing a Le Fort II type fracture with dental injuries. (Reproduced with kind permission of Springer Science+Business Media.)

Imaging for specific facial fractures

Fractures of the mandible (including condylar fractures)

Panoral tomography

A panoral tomogram, or othopantomogram (OPT), represents the best single overall view of the mandible, including an excellent view of the condyles. The combination of a postero-anterior (PA) view of the mandible and a panoral tomogram usually obviates the need for further radiographs in most patients and significantly reduces the overall radiation dose to the patient.

A commonly taught principle in trauma radiology is to obtain at least two views, each taken at right angles to the other, in order to assess the degree of displacement and angulation of the fragments. With the mandible this is often thought to be achieved by taking an OPT and a PA view. However, the views of the symphyseal region in both these views are in reality quite similar, and certainly not at 90°. The cervical spine is also superimposed on the symphysis in an OPT and can obscure detailed assessment. If uncertainty exists in this region a lower occlusal view is a useful additional image (Fig. 4.2).

If panoral tomography is unavailable, left and right oblique lateral views in combination with a rotated PA projection can be substituted (Fig. 4.3).

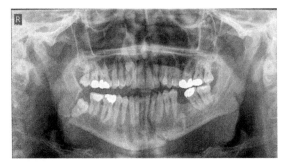

Figure 4.2 A correctly taken othopantomogram gives an excellent image of the whole mandible from condyle to condyle, although the clarity of the anterior region may be affected by the overlying shadow of the cervical spine. Accurate assessment of the dental status requires additional intraoral radiographs.

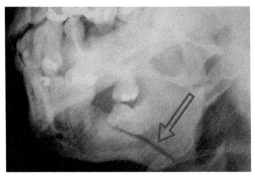

Figure 4.3 An oblique lateral radiograph of the mandible may occasionally be helpful to image a suspected fracture of the mandible, although this is normally indicated only where an OPT is unavailable. (Reproduced with kind permission of Springer Science+Business Media.)

Postero-anterior (PA) and antero-posterior (AP) projections

The standard PA view of the face, with the central ray angled 10° upwards to the horizontal radiographic base line, demonstrates fractures of the body and angle together with the degree of displacement in the sagittal plane (Fig. 4.4). Combining it with an OPT, which essentially adds the lateral view, provides the best overall assessment of mandibular fractures using plain radiographs alone.

Although the PA view is also useful for imaging most condylar neck fractures the condylar head may be obscured by superimposition of the skull base and mastoid process. For this reason, and if the OPT needs supplementing with additional information in a sagittal

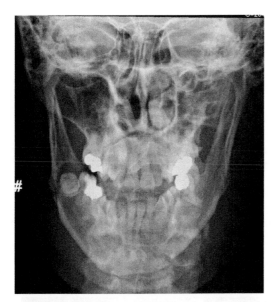

Figure 4.4 Postero-anterior radiograph showing a fracture of the right angle and anterior region of the mandible. The overlying shadow of the cervical spine obscures accurate assessment of the anterior region. If this is still unclear on an OPT a rotated PA view and/or occlusal view may be indicated.

plane, the 30° antero-posterior Townes projection is sometimes used. This view demonstrates the condylar region very well, along with the posterior fossa of the skull. In order to avoid changing the position of the patient who has had an OM or PA view taken, a reverse Townes projection may be used to achieve the same effect although it is less satisfactory. In both projections the central ray is angled at 30° to the horizontal base line, which throws the image of the condylar head and subcondylar region clear of the dense bony structures of the base of the skull.

Intra-oral radiographs

Periapical views are ideal for the most accurate assessment of the teeth and their relationship to the line of fracture, although too often this is decided entirely from the OPT. Occlusal views across the fracture line may help to evaluate the relationship of a dental root to the fracture, and are also invaluable for demonstrating midline fractures of the mandible with minimal displacement. Oblique fractures are also well demonstrated. Anterior occlusal views can also identify avulsion-type fractures of the lingual plate or genial tubercles, although CT may be preferable.

CT and MRI

CT offers very little advantage as a diagnostic tool in simple injuries of the lower third of the face and is not normally undertaken for isolated mandibular fractures unless there are complicating factors such as significant comminution. In this situation the construction of a three-dimensional model may be helpful to facilitate pre-surgical planning and the pre-bending of a rigid reconstruction plate.

CT is also useful in the assessment of displaced and comminuted fractures of the condylar region where it will demonstrate considerable detail that would otherwise not be clear on standard radiographs, such as an undisplaced vertical fracture of the condylar head (Fig. 4.5).

Magnetic resonance imaging may visualize the meniscus within the temporomandibular joint and

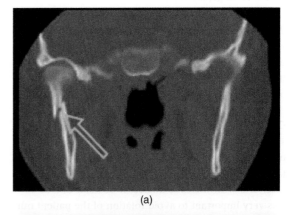

(a)

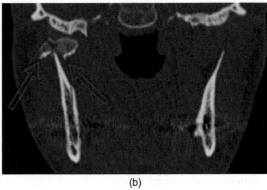

(b)

Figure 4.5 Coronal CT scans showing (a) overriding fracture of right condylar neck and (b) comminuted fracture of right condylar head. (Reproduced with kind permission of Springer Science+Business Media.)

demonstrate the presence of effusions, but this is rarely required as an urgent investigation.

Le Fort type midface fractures

The complexity of imaging required to obtain a detailed picture of a midfacial fracture needs to be balanced against the benefits to actual treatment planning. Not every midface fractures requires a CT scan. For example, separation at the Le Fort I level can often be ascertained as a clinical diagnosis alone, although plain radiographs at least are advised. At this level intraoral views are invaluable in assessing associated dentoalveolar injuries or in confirming a midline split of the palate, both factors that have a major influence on treatment. For higher level Le Fort II and III type fractures, it is important to determine the overall fracture pattern and particularly the degree of cranial and orbital involvement.

True lateral projection

Le Fort type fractures at each level (I, II and III) can be detected on this view where the fracture line can be seen passing across the pterygoid plates. It is often the only plain view that clearly demonstrates a Le Fort I fracture. It also aids recognition and assessment of any extension of fractures into the frontal sinus.

Occipitomental projection

The occipitomental (OM) view is the single most useful plain radiograph in midfacial trauma. Two projections taken in the correct postero-anterior position are desirable, one with the tube angled at 10° and one at 30°. It is very important to avoid rotation of the patient out of the sagittal plane. These views will demonstrate most uncomplicated midfacial fractures with sufficient detail to determine a treatment plan. However, in higher level trauma, a CT scan is often advisable in addition in order to visualize the orbital walls and orbital apex. With plain views fractures are only clearly visible where bone is thick, or where thin bone plates lie at a tangent to the X-ray beam.

Due to the combination of complex anatomy, superimposition of the skull base and the relatively unusual angle of the views compared to images taken in conventional anatomical planes, interpretation of OM radiographs can be challenging for the inexperienced clinician. These views need to be examined systematically along lines where bone disjunction can be expected if a midface fracture has occurred. To help

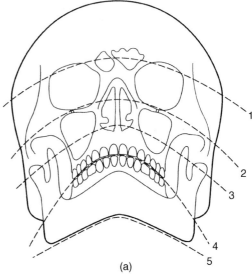

(a)

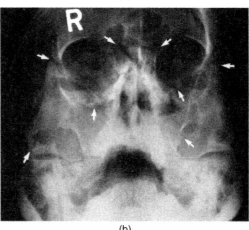

(b)

Figure 4.6 (a) Diagram to show the four search lines (Campbell's lines) that can be systematically followed as an aid in interpreting occipitomental radiographs. The fifth line was described later by Trapnell. (b) OM radiograph of patient with Le Fort II and III type fractures. The arrows denote fracture sites which lie on Campbell's lines.

this, four curved search lines, referred to as Campbell's lines, are frequently used (Fig. 4.6). A fifth line that follows the lower border of the mandible was suggested later by Trapnell.

CT imaging

If a midface maxillary fracture is clearly more complex, with significant comminution and displacement, then the detailed information provided by CT is required

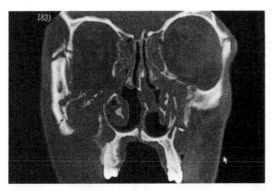

Figure 4.7 Coronal CT scan of a complex midface fracture demonstrating the comminution which may not be immediately obvious on plain radiographs. Note the midline split of the palate.

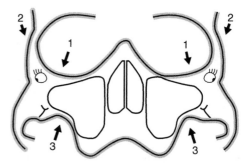

Figure 4.8 The 'elephant's head' approach to the assessment of zygomatic fractures. Fracture lines are commonly seen at (1) the infraorbital rim, (2) the frontozygomatic suture region, (3) the lateral wall of the maxillary antrum (zygomatic buttress) and the zygomatic arch ('trunk'). (Reproduced with kind permission of Elsevier.)

in order to determine the surgical risks and plan the repair (Fig. 4.7). It is particularly important to determine whether or not a fracture involves the anterior skull base (Le Fort II and III levels) since manipulation of fractures extending into this area may result in dural tears.

Fractures of the zygomatic complex
Occipitomental projection
As with Le Fort type fractures, two OM projections (10° and 30°) will generally delineate the fracture pattern and displacement of the zygomatic complex, including isolated fractures of the zygomatic arch. Careful interpretation using Campbell's lines will help identify the fracture sites and determine any asymmetry, which can sometimes be quite subtle. A number of other approaches have been described to help in the interpretation of OM views, including imagining the zygomatic complex as an 'elephant's head' and searching for abnormalities at the common fracture sites (Fig. 4.8). A trap for the inexperienced clinician is to assume that the fronto-zygomatic suture represents a fracture line, particularly if it is very obvious.

CT imaging
CT scans are sometimes indicated in zygomatic fractures, particularly where there is extensive associated damage to the orbital floor, concomitant expansion of the orbital volume or comminution of the zygomatic bone and arch. Occasionally impaction of the zygomatic complex can produce compression of the orbit with proptosis (Fig. 4.9). More precise definition of such an injury, which includes the possibility of globe rupture,

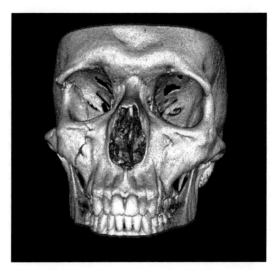

Figure 4.9 Three-dimensional CT image of an impacted fracture of the right zygomatic complex. Note particularly the medial displacement at the frontozygomatic suture region. (Reproduced with kind permission of Springer Science+Business Media.)

is then desirable by means of CT. 'Telescoping' or fragmentation of the zygomatic arch will usually require wide exposure and open reduction to restore midface width and projection. In this situation CT is preferable to the alternative plain submento-vertex view.

Isolated orbital floor ('blowout') fractures
The characteristic feature of the isolated orbital floor fracture is the absence of obvious bony damage to the zygomatic complex, even though clinical examination

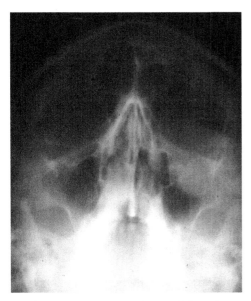

Figure 4.10 'Hanging drop' sign. The rounded opacity seen in the left maxillary antrum is due to herniation of orbital contents following an isolated fracture of the left orbital floor ('blow-out' fracture).

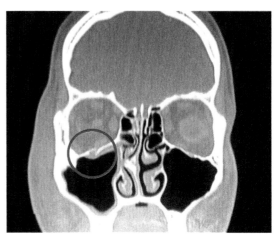

Figure 4.11 Coronal CT scan of a patient with clinical signs of tethering of the right inferior rectus following orbital injury. This subtle evidence of an isolated orbital floor fracture would not be seen on a plain radiograph. (Reproduced with kind permission of Springer Science+Business Media.)

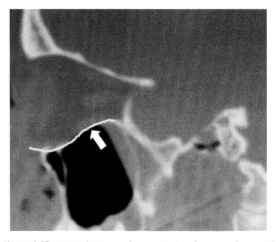

Figure 4.12 Coronal CT scan demonstrating the normal sigmoid outline of the orbital floor giving a so-called 'posteromedial bulge'. Orbital floor fractures frequently involve this area with loss of contour. Accurate identification of the defect and restoration of this shape is essential if secondary enophthalmos is to be minimized. (See also Fig. 3.20.)

may suggest the presence of such an injury. The classical 'hanging drop' appearance of a large orbital floor defect with herniation of orbital contents is usually first noted in the OM projection (Fig. 4.10). However, this is not a reliable sign since blood clot and a mucus retention cyst in the sinus can both present with similar radiological features. In fact, plain radiographs of isolated orbital floor fractures are not required unless there is suspected bony injury elsewhere. Plain radiographs may incidentally show evidence of orbital floor or wall fractures, but are notoriously unreliable in excluding such an injury or determining its extent.

Any decision to investigate further should be based on clinical assessment. Both CT and MRI can give useful information, but CT has the advantage of better bone visualization and more widespread availability (Fig. 4.11). With appropriate software CT can also be used to predict whether enophthalmos will occur, and its extent if the injury is untreated. Enophthalmos is more likely to develop where there is loss of the 'posteromedial bulge' of the orbital floor, best seen in sagittal views (Fig. 4.12). The posterior limit of the defect also gives an indication of difficulty when it comes to repair.

If access to CT is unavailable, plain tomography or ultrasound examination are alternative methods of investigation, which can be used to confirm the presence of a blow-out fracture with an indication of its extent.

Naso-orbito-ethmoid fractures

These fractures vary considerably in their complexity. Plain radiographs provide insufficient detail of damage to the medial orbital walls, nasal septum and floor of the anterior cranial fossa to enable operative repair to be planned with confidence. CT scans on the other hand provide a much more complete picture and are an essential investigation for the accurate assessment of this type of injury.

Frontal bone and craniofacial fractures

Fractures of the upper third are usually primarily a frontal bone injury with coincidental involvement of the midfacial skeleton. There is often associated damage to the brain or meninges. Rupture of the dura with leakage of CSF into the nasal or orbital cavity can occur. There may be other concomitant intracranial injuries including extradural and intra-cerebral haematomas, traumatic encephalocoele and pneumocephalus. The frontal sinuses are often involved and it is important to know whether fractures extend into the posterior wall or orbital roof where the dura may be perforated or torn. It is also important to assess involvement of the frontonasal duct in the fracture pattern. Such an injury, if mistreated can lead to delayed mucocoele or empyema formation. Pre-operative diagnosis of these types of severe injuries can only be made with confidence from CT and MRI scans.

Further reading

Karjodkar JR. *Textbook of Dental and Maxillofacial Radiology.* Jaypee Brothers; Medical Publishers; 2008.

McDonald D. *Oral and Maxillofacial Radiology: A Diagnostic Approach.* Wiley-Blackwell; 2011.

CHAPTER 5

Treatment of dentoalveolar injuries

The term 'dentoalveolar injury' describes trauma that is localized to the teeth and the supporting structures of the alveolus. These injuries can occur in isolation, or as part of a more serious maxillofacial injury. Isolated dentoalveolar injuries usually follow relatively minor accidents, such as falls or collisions during sport or play. The majority of patients presenting with isolated dentoalveolar injuries are children or adolescents and, as might be expected, boys are at much greater risk than girls. Despite the use of mouth guards in many sporting activities these injuries are still common. Cycling accidents and minor road traffic accidents are a common cause. Injury to the teeth can sometimes occur during epileptic seizures, and iatrogenic damage may take place during extraction of ankylosed teeth, endoscopy procedures or endotracheal intubation. The possibility of non-accidental injury should always be borne in mind, particularly in younger children.

Depending on local arrangements, these injuries may be managed by hospital clinics, specialist dental practitioners or the patient's own dentist. Whatever the arrangements, long-term follow-up is required because some complications can occur months, or even years, later. Most dentoalveolar injuries can be treated in the primary dental care setting under local analgesia, particularly in those cases where damage is limited to the teeth without alveolar fracture.

Dentoalveolar injuries are among the very few fractures of the facial skeleton where immediate treatment is important. Obvious or suspected exposures of the dental pulp require early treatment, not only for the relief of pain but also to ensure the best prognosis. Whereas simple jaw fractures are rarely very painful, injuries to vital teeth can cause severe pain compounded by any associated interference with the occlusion. Unfortunately the level of knowledge and expertise required for the emergency and ongoing treatment of dental trauma is sometimes lacking in general dental practice, and even in the hospital setting the initial management of the dental component of a facial injury is often far from ideal.

Classification

A comprehensive classification of dentoalveolar injuries and full details of the management of damaged teeth are outside the scope of this book. Many excellent specialist texts on the subject exist and should be consulted for further information (see Further reading at the end of the chapter). Table 5.1 gives a descriptive classification of dentoalveolar injuries, which is also illustrated in Figs. 5.1, 5.2 and 5.3.

The pattern and complexity of a dentoalveolar injury depends on a number of factors. These include the site and energy of impact, the strength of the teeth, the resilience of the periodontal structures and the elasticity of the alveolar bone. The latter two factors in particular are related to the age of the patient and the presence or otherwise of pre-existing periodontal disease. Single or multiple teeth can be damaged individually, or a complete segment of alveolar bone can be fractured with relatively little damage to the group of teeth it supports. Table 5.2 summarizes the typical clinical findings following different types of injury.

Clinical assessment

Injuries to the teeth occur in approximately one third of fractures affecting the tooth bearing areas of the jaws. Therefore, both components need careful assessment. Fortunately the vast majority of dental or dentoalveolar injuries are relatively minor and occur in isolation,

Fractures of the Facial Skeleton, Second Edition. Michael Perry, Andrew Brown and Peter Banks.
© 2015 John Wiley & Sons, Ltd. Published 2015 by John Wiley & Sons, Ltd.

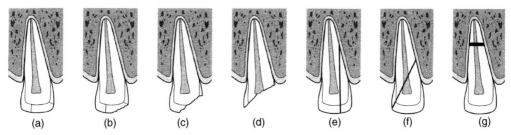

Figure 5.1 Injuries to the dental hard tissues and pulp as classified in Table 5.1. (a) Crown infraction. (b) Enamel fracture. (c) Enamel + dentine fracture. (d) Enamel + dentine + pulp fracture. (e) Vertical crown-root fracture. (f) Oblique crown-root fracture. (g) Root fracture.

Table 5.1 Classification of dentoalveolar injuries.

1 Dental hard tissue injury (see Fig. 5.1)
   a. Crown infraction (crack of enamel or incomplete fracture)
   b. Crown fracture – Enamel only
   c. Crown fracture – Enamel + dentine
   d. Crown fracture – Enamel + dentine + pulp
   e. Crown – root fracture (vertical fracture)
   f. Crown – root fracture (oblique fracture)
   g. Root fracture
2 Periodontal injury (see Fig. 5.2)
   a. Concussion (no displacement of tooth but tender to percussion)
   b. Subluxation (loosening of tooth without displacement)
   c. Intrusion
   d. Extrusion
   e. Lateral luxation (loosening of tooth with displacement)
   f. Avulsion
3 Alveolar bone injury (see Fig. 5.3)|
   a. Intrusion of tooth with comminution of socket
   b. Fracture of single wall of socket or alveolus
   c. Fracture of both walls of socket or alveolus
   d. Fracture of mandible or maxilla involving the alveolus and/or tooth socket
4 Gingival injury
   a. Contusion
   b. Abrasion
   c. Laceration
5 Combinations of the above

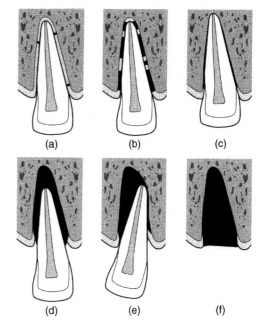

Figure 5.2 Injuries involving the periodontal tissues as classified in Table 5.1. (a) Concussion. (b) Subluxation. (c) Intrusion. (d) Extrusion. (e) Lateral luxation. (f) Avulsion.

often involving only a single tooth and its periodontal membrane. Nevertheless correct management is important to avoid later discolouration or loss of teeth, both of which can have a major aesthetic impact. A thorough clinical assessment of the dentition requires a good light, adequate retraction of the lips and cheeks, a fine tipped sucker, the use of a dental mirror and probe and a cooperative patient. These conditions are normally achievable with a conscious adult but in the case of a distressed young child full assessment may require sedation or a general anaesthetic.

Dental fractures

The type of dental fracture seen is usually related to the mechanism of injury. Anterior teeth are commonly fractured by direct impact and there is often an associated ragged laceration of the inner surface of the upper lip, or a laceration in the buccal sulcus with partial degloving of the soft tissues. Injury to the posterior dentition, with vertical splitting of one or more teeth, may result from forceful impaction of the two jaws

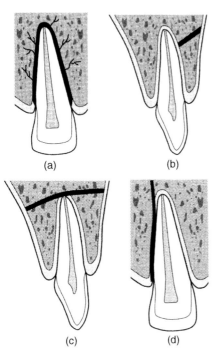

(a)   (b)

(c)   (d)

Figure 5.3 Injuries of the alveolar bone as classified in Table 5.1. (a) Comminution of socket. (b) Fracture of one socket wall. (c) Fracture of either both socket walls or alveolus. (d) Fracture of jaw involving socket.

Table 5.2 Clinical findings following different types of dentoalveolar injury.

Type of injury	Pattern of injury
a. Force distributed over several teeth, or impact cushioned by overlying soft tissues	Concussion
	Subluxation
	Lateral luxation
	Intrusion
	Alveolar segmental fracture
b. Direct force to teeth	Crown fracture
	Root fracture
	Displacement of teeth or avulsion
	Penetrating lip wounds
c. Indirect force to teeth (e.g. axial blow to chin)	Crown-root fracture (vertical split)
	Possible associated jaw fracture (including split maxilla)

together. This can occur in association with a number of relatively minor injuries including anterior flexion of the neck as part of a 'whiplash' type injury. In such cases the jaws themselves may remain relatively uninjured. Meticulous dental examination is therefore essential, including percussion of the teeth and careful probing of the crowns. Any missing fragments of crown or missing fillings should be noted.

Subluxation and displacement of teeth usually causes derangement of the occlusion. Fragments of teeth may become embedded in lip or tongue lacerations, or they may be swallowed. Only rarely are they inhaled, but this should always be considered, especially if there has been a history of loss of consciousness. Individual teeth may also be missing and an empty tooth socket clearly suggests that the tooth concerned has been knocked out. If a tooth or fragment of tooth cannot be accounted for a chest radiograph should be ordered, plus ideally a soft tissue view of the neck. Where missing teeth are noted it is important to be sure no retained roots are present.

Fractures of the roots of teeth may be difficult to diagnose clinically. Excessively mobile teeth that do not appear to be subluxed are suspect and should be noted for later periapical radiographs. Occasionally molar and premolar teeth appear superficially normal but close inspection reveals either a vertical split or a horizontal fracture just below the gingival margin.

Vitality testing soon after injury, whether electrical or thermal, is unreliable and of little use in determining the eventual prognosis for the pulp. This is because a blow of sufficient force to disrupt the alveolus will usually disturb the function of the nerve endings supplying individual teeth whose blood supply may nevertheless be intact.

Alveolar fractures

Alveolar fractures in the mandible are frequently associated with fractures of the jaw itself, whereas in the maxilla they are more often isolated injuries. Occasionally there may be evidence of a fractured alveolus with no associated injury to the teeth themselves. However, intact teeth within a fractured alveolar segment should be presumed to have been devitalized until evidence to the contrary emerges during the period of follow-up. Severe trauma to either jaw may result in gross comminution of the alveolus, but more often an alveolar fracture consists of one or two distinct fragments containing teeth (Fig. 5.4). During the initial examination it may be possible gently to reposition loose alveolar fragments and the earlier this is achieved the better the prognosis for individual teeth.

In severe comminuted lower jaw fractures a complete alveolar fragment may be displaced into the soft

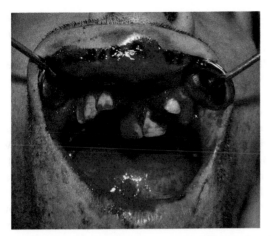

Figure 5.4 Maxillary dentoalveolar injury. The luxated central incisors have been displaced posteriorly with their fractured supporting bone, causing associated vertical lacerations of the fixed gingivae. There is also a laceration on the inner surface of the upper lip due to the impact.

tissues of the floor of the mouth and can on occasions appear completely covered by mucosa. In the symphyseal region it may be difficult to determine clinically whether such a loose alveolar segment is actually part of a complete fracture of the mandible or not.

Maxillary alveolar fractures occur most often in the incisor region in which case there may be obvious deformity of the alveolus and disturbance of the occlusion. This is not always the case as some fractured segments can be impacted into the relatively soft bone of the maxilla and become virtually immobile. Where clinical examination reveals damage to teeth or bruising of the alveolar mucosa, careful palpation is necessary to exclude any underlying alveolar fracture. Sometimes crepitation can be detected on palpation and a 'cracked pot' note detected when the teeth within the fractured alveolus are percussed.

Fracture of the maxillary tuberosity and fracture of the antral floor are recognized complications of upper molar extractions (see Fig. 5.8), and in one sense a midline split of the palate converts a Le Fort I fracture into two large dentoalveolar segments.

The radiographic examination of dentoalveolar injuries must include occlusal and/or periapical dental radiographs. With the widespread use of panoral tomography these views are perhaps less used than they should be in the diagnosis of maxillofacial trauma, but full assessment of injuries to the teeth is impossible without them.

Associated soft tissue injuries

Displacement of a dentoalveolar fragment is usually associated with a vertical split laceration of the overlying fixed gingiva and anterior dentoalveolar fractures are commonly associated with significant damage to the lips. There is often substantial bruising and swelling and there may be portions of tooth or foreign bodies embedded in the soft tissues. Inspection may reveal a full thickness perforating wound of one or other lip, or a ragged laceration on the inner aspect, both caused by impaction against the anterior teeth.

Dentoalveolar fractures in the anterior region of the mandible can sometimes be associated with a 'degloving' injury that results from impaction of the point of the chin on some resilient surface such as soft earth. The jaw itself does not fracture but the soft tissue is rotated violently over the point of the chin and a horizontal tear occurs in the labial sulcus at the junction of the attached and free gingiva.

Treatment

Dental trauma frequently requires immediate treatment, both to relieve pain and often to preserve the dentition. Early treatment is imperative if there is exposure or near exposure of the pulp chamber or subluxation of an individual tooth or teeth. The dental injury will often therefore take precedence over most other facial bone fractures. When a dentoalveolar fracture occurs in isolation, the injury is easily recognized and effective treatment is usually offered immediately. However, when damage to individual teeth is part of a more extensive facial injury, the importance of early intervention may be forgotten. Treatment of dental injuries should have the same priority as the treatment of facial lacerations. Simple measures such as repositioning of displaced teeth and protection of the pulp are sometimes overlooked in the initial management of a complex facial injury. In an unconscious multiply injured patient requiring endotracheal intubation stabilization of any loose teeth or alveolar segments will minimize difficulties in repositioning the tube and prevent further dental damage. Similarly, covering or extirpating the exposed dental pulp will reduce the painful stimuli that can contribute to restlessness in the unconscious patient. Of course all these measures need to be undertaken at an appropriate time, depending on the clinical status of the patient.

In the comprehensive treatment planning of den-toalveolar injuries, several factors have to be taken into consideration. The relative importance of preserving damaged teeth will vary according to the complexity of the maxillofacial injury, the age of the patient, the general dental condition including oral hygiene, periodontal disease and crowding, the site and extent of the dentoalveolar injury and the wishes of the patient. The prognosis for traumatized teeth and the healing of alveolar fractures are generally better in younger patients. Smoking and poor oral hygiene significantly increase the risks of infection and loss of teeth. Open root apices, intact gingival tissues, absence of root fractures and good periodontal bone support are all clinical conditions that are indicative of a favourable outcome.

In the deciduous dentition the pattern of injury differs from adolescents and adults because the elasticity and thinness of the alveolar bone usually protects and prevents fracture of the dentition. Segmental fractures of the alveolus are extremely rare for the same reason. The more complex dentoalveolar injuries normally involve the permanent dentition. In planning treatment it is best to consider each tooth in turn using the classification outlined here (Table 5.1). Injuries to any particular patient may range from a small chip off a cusp or incisal edge to multiple broken and displaced teeth with an associated fracture of the supporting alveolus.

Injuries to the primary dentition

Approximately 70% of injuries to the primary dentition involve the maxillary central incisors. Intrusion and lateral luxation are the commonest injury with avulsion occurring in approximately 10% of cases. Generally speaking, fractured, extruded or grossly displaced teeth should be extracted. Less displaced teeth that do not cause occlusal interference can be left and monitored. Damage to the underlying developing permanent tooth germ by displaced teeth is a commonly recognized problem, particularly with intrusion injuries. Intruded primary teeth will usually re-erupt spontaneously and attempted extraction of a deeply intruded tooth simply increases the risk of further damage to underlying permanent tooth germs.

Injuries affecting the permanent dentition

As newer dental materials become available, the com-prehensive management of dental trauma will no doubt continue to evolve. What follows is therefore an overview, focusing on the early stages of care. An up to date text on the subject should be consulted for fuller details of current management. Guidelines and protocols now exist for many of these injuries.

Injuries to the dental hard tissue
Crown fracture

Fractures of the crown may involve the enamel only (Fig 5.1b); enamel and dentine (Fig. 5.1c); or enamel, dentine and pulp (Fig. 5.1d). All injured teeth should be radiographed to exclude subgingival fractures.

A simple chip or fracture of the enamel only does not require emergency treatment. These teeth are usually slightly tender and may not have any obvious signs of injury. Cracks may be visible using a bright light to tran-silluminate the crown, with a blue light being particu-larly useful. Cracks can be sealed with an appropriate bonding agent or composite material.

Any exposure of dentine should be covered as soon as possible, particularly in young people where bacterial penetration of the open dentinal tubules can be rapid. The tooth is typically tender to touch and is sensitive on exposure to the air or hot and cold liquids. A small yellow patch of dentine may be visible. After gently cleaning, protection with a calcium hydroxide cement, held in place with a temporary acid-etch composite dressing is ideal until a definitive restoration can be undertaken. Providing it is large enough, considera-tion can be given to restoring the fractured crown by cementing the fragment with composite resin. Pulp testing immediately after injury is of no clinical value, but the tooth must be carefully followed up and root treated later if necessary.

If the pulp is exposed it is not only exquisitely painful to touch and thermal stimuli but will also eventually necrose. Small exposures treated early can be managed as earlier and monitored, but larger exposures or delays in treatment will require a pulpotomy and calcium hydroxide dressing if the apex is still open, or pulp extirpation if the apex is closed.

Root fracture

An oblique fracture of the crown may extend subgin-givally as a crown-root fracture (Figs. 5.1e and 5.1f). In this situation a decision has to be taken about the possi-bility of saving the tooth following the same emergency methods described previously. Successful long-term results depend on establishing a good seal of both the fracture line and the pulp cavity. If the fracture extends a considerable way down the root, or if there is a vertical split and the crown is very mobile, extraction is likely.

Transverse fractures of the root (Fig. 5.1g) usually affect the incisor teeth and the prognosis depends to a large extent on the level of fracture. A calcified or fibrous bridge occasionally results in 'healing' of the root, particularly if the fracture is in the apical third, but fractures that occur near the gingival level have a poorer prognosis. If the tooth is to be conserved it should be rigidly splinted for at least 6 weeks. It can be immobilized by bonding to adjacent teeth with acid etch composite, or a wire and acid-etch composite splint can be applied.

Pulp necrosis, root resorption and obliteration of the pulp canal are common consequences of root fracture, occurring in up to 60% of cases. In fractures that lay close to the gingival margin the tooth can sometimes still be restored following endodontic treatment and orthodontic extrusion or a crown lengthening procedure. However, extraction and an osseointegrated implant is likely to be the preferred option in many cases.

Injuries to the periodontal tissues
Luxation
Luxation, or loosening of a tooth, requires a short period of splintage with occlusal adjustment to relieve any interference. Pulp haemorrhage can occur following simple concussion of a tooth and any loosening or displacement carries a high risk of subsequent pulp necrosis, particularly following intrusion injuries. As with root fractures additional late complications include root resorption, pulp canal obliteration, ankylosis and loss of marginal bone support.

Teeth that have been loosened, laterally luxated or extruded should be manipulated back into position and splinted for 7–21 days (see Table 5.3). If a semi-rigid splint is indicated a piece of light wire or orthodontic wire is bonded with acid-etch composite to the splint the damaged tooth to adjacent sound teeth.

If acid-etch composite materials are not available soft stainless steel wire can sometimes be used to construct a splint. A loop of wire is passed around a group of teeth, incorporating one or two teeth distal to the subluxed teeth. Individual tie wires are then passed interdentally and tightened to take up the slack in the loop and immobilize the loose teeth (Fig. 5.5). Simple splints for subluxed teeth or minor alveolar fractures

Table 5.3 Types of splint and suggested duration of treatment in dentoalveolar injuries.

Injury	Splint	Duration of splinting
Root fracture	Rigid	6 weeks minimum
Extrusion	Semi-rigid	7–10 days
Lateral luxation	Semi-rigid	2–3 weeks
Avulsion	Semi-rigid	7–10 days
Alveolar fracture		
Block segment of teeth	Rigid	4–6 weeks
Fracture of labial/lingual plate	Semi-rigid	4–6 weeks

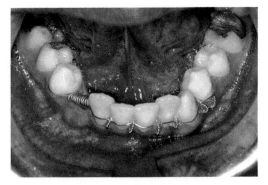

Figure 5.5 Subluxed lower incisors immobilized by a simple soft wire loop splint with interdental tie wires.

can also be constructed from vacuum-formed plastic. An impression is taken following repositioning of the tooth or alveolar fragment. A thin plastic veneer splint is then vacuum-formed in the laboratory. The splint can be self-retaining but is usually fixed with a zinc oxide based cement or cold-cure acrylic resin (Fig. 5.6), although individually chipped or fractured teeth should be covered with calcium hydroxide as described earlier. A criticism of cemented splints of this type is that they may compromise oral hygiene leading to gingival inflammation and interference with healing of the traumatized tissues.

Avulsion
Avulsion (exarticulation) is the complete separation of the tooth from its socket. This is an urgent situation requiring immediate action. A number of factors influence the chance of success following replantation

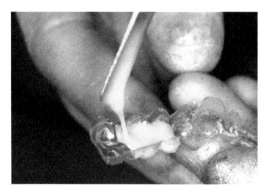

Figure 5.6 Thin vacuum-formed plastic splint being filled with cold-cure acrylic resin prior to cementation for stabilization of loose teeth.

of an avulsed tooth. These include the stage of root development, the length of time the tooth is allowed to dry, the length of storage outside the mouth, the medium used and correct handling and splinting. Immediate replacement is still the ideal treatment. If the tooth is put back almost immediately (i.e. within the first 5 minutes) there is a good chance of success. However, if this is delayed more than 2 hours, the prognosis for survival is poor. The first priority is therefore to replant any avulsed adult tooth as soon as possible.

Ideally the root should not be handled to avoid damage to the periodontal ligament cells, but some damage is inevitable if the tooth has been retrieved from a playground or sports field. Debris should be removed by gentle rinsing for a few seconds under running cold water. Once the tooth is replaced the patient should bite gently on a handkerchief or gauze and an emergency appointment should be made with a dental surgeon for semi-rigid splinting.

If the tooth cannot be replanted immediately it is important to ensure that the cells of the periodontal ligament do not dry out. Survival out of the mouth is possible for up to 30 minutes but few cells will retain any vitality after 60 minutes. However, it has been shown that periodontal cells will retain their vitality for 2 hours in the patient's own saliva and 6 hours in fresh milk. Water is a harmful storage medium due to osmotic lysis of the cells.

Provided that the tooth is kept moist in milk it may be possible to replant it up to 24 hours later. If the tooth has been dry for 20–60 minutes, some authorities recommend first soaking it in a balanced salt solution for 30 minutes. If it has been dry for more than 60 minutes

it has been suggested to first soak it in citric acid for five minutes, then in 2% stannous fluoride for 10 minutes, and finally in doxycycline for five minutes before reimplantation is attempted. This has been reported to reduce root resorption and increase the likelihood of success. Some studies have shown that when a tooth has been out of the mouth for longer than 60 minutes, immediate reimplantation is no longer critical. Root canal therapy can therefore be performed on the tooth before it is put back in the socket. Long term survival will always be unpredictable.

Curettage of the socket should be avoided because it is associated with increased resorption. It should instead be irrigated with warm saline to clear any clot or debris. The tooth is held by the crown and the root gently irrigated to wash off the storage medium. It is then firmly replanted in the socket. The alveolus should be compressed to reduce any fracture of the socket wall. A semi-rigid splint is applied for 7–14 days and a course of antibiotics prescribed.

Even if the eventual outlook is poor it is still worth attempting to save a tooth in the short term since this will help alveolar healing and will retain alveolar bone in the area, which is an important factor if a dental implant is to be considered at a later date.

Injuries to the alveolar bone

Alveolar fractures involving a block of alveolar bone, or sometimes the labial and lingual socket walls, usually occur in the anterior or premolar region. The commonest posterior fracture is an iatrogenic fracture of the maxillary tuberosity that may complicate the extraction of upper molar teeth. As with other facial fractures the treatment of displaced alveolar fractures involves reduction and fixation. Closed reduction of the alveolar segment is usually achieved by finger manipulation and a suitable splint is then applied. Care needs to be taken to avoid displacing the loose teeth during the reduction and any splint used must extend to enough sound teeth to achieve satisfactory immobilization. Open reduction is rarely performed in alveolar fractures unless access is required as part of the treatment of an underlying jaw fracture.

A rigid wire and composite splint is effective in the anterior region (Fig. 5.7) but is more difficult to apply in the posterior maxillary arch. Arch bars and interdental wiring have the drawback of being more traumatic to the gingival tissues and there is a risk of avulsing loose

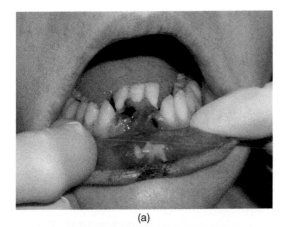

(a)

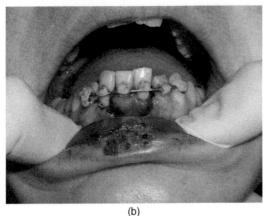

(b)

Figure 5.7 (a) Dentoalveolar fracture in which a block of alveolar bone containing three lower incisors has been displaced posteriorly. (b) Reduction of the fractured segment and fixation with a heavy wire splint bonded to the displaced teeth and to sound teeth either side. Excellent oral hygiene needs to be maintained to promote uncomplicated healing of the contused and lacerated gingivae. (Reproduced with kind permission of Springer Science+Business Media.)

teeth as the wires are tightened. The individual teeth in the alveolar fragment need to be examined carefully and treated appropriately if damaged. A minor problem occurs occasionally with isolated displaced alveolar fractures in that it is sometimes difficult to avoid leaving the teeth slightly 'high' after reduction. This results in premature contact and continuing trauma to the teeth. The occlusion needs to be checked carefully and the bite adjusted if necessary. Occasionally a short period of intermaxillary fixation is a sensible precaution, particularly if the fragment is very mobile.

Comminuted fractures of the alveolus in the incisor area, with or without comminution of associated teeth, usually necessitate the removal of the portions of teeth and alveolus and careful soft-tissue repair of the resulting alveolar defect. All portions of alveolar bone that appear to have a chance of survival should be preserved. Lacerated wounds of the lip should be carefully explored and irrigated, and any fragments of teeth removed. The edges of the wound can then be minimally trimmed if necessary and closure carried out.

Extraction of damaged teeth from a block of fractured alveolus should be avoided if at all possible. Unless an extremely careful surgical technique is used there is a significant risk of tearing the mucosal attachment and avulsing the whole segment. Ideally any surgical extraction of teeth or roots should be delayed for 6–8 weeks when bone healing will be advanced and the mucoperiosteal tissues healthy.

This principle applies to fractures of the maxillary tuberosity. This complication often results because of ankylosis or root bulbosity affecting the maxillary molar teeth. The thin supporting alveolar bone and antral floor fractures on attempted forceps extraction. The operator becomes aware that a whole dentoalveolar block extending to the tuberosity is mobile on moving the tooth. On occasion the palatal mucoperiosteum tears longitudinally as a result of the forcible buccal movement with the extraction forceps. If the tuberosity is essentially detached from the periosteum it should be carefully dissected out and the resulting soft-tissue defect repaired to minimize any subsequent communication with the maxillary sinus (Fig. 5.8).

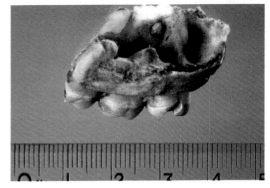

Figure 5.8 Dentoalveolar fracture of maxillary alveolus and tuberosity as a result of attempted extraction of ankylosed teeth with bulbous roots. The fragment has been dissected free prior to repair of the resulting oro-antral communication.

If the tuberosity, with or without associated teeth, appears to be well attached to the periosteum, it can be left alone with or without splinting. Splinting of the tooth attached to the fragment with fixation to other standing teeth in the maxilla for 4–6 weeks usually results in union. A simple way to achieve this is to fabricate a full coverage palatal acrylic plate that should extend around the palatal surfaces of the affected teeth. The splint can be retained by Adams cribs, including one or more engaging the mobile segment.

If the tooth in the tuberosity fragment requires extraction it should be removed surgically once the tuberosity is firm. If the tooth is painful, this surgical extraction may have to be carried out earlier, but the chance of saving the tuberosity in such circumstances is greatly reduced.

Other fractures extending to the alveolar floor of the maxillary sinus are treated in the same way, depending upon whether the alveolar fragment, together with any associated teeth, is completely detached from the periosteum. Should a portion of alveolus and floor of the antrum be inadvertently removed during the extraction of a tooth a very careful soft-tissue repair of the defect must be carried out immediately, if necessary by advancing a buccal mucoperiosteal flap with or without a buccal fat flap. The patient should avoid nose blowing and should be prescribed a nasal decongestant and a short course of antibiotics to prevent infection causing breakdown and development of an oro-antral fistula.

Injuries to the gingivae

Most dentoalveolar injuries are associated with some degree of gingival damage. The maintenance of good gingival health is important for uncomplicated healing, and will improve the outcome for replanted or replaced teeth. A suitable antiseptic mouthwash should be prescribed in the postoperative period.

Displacement of teeth or a block of alveolar bone is commonly associated with small vertical gingival lacerations (Fig. 5.7b). These usually heal well following reduction of the fracture and rarely need suturing. If a piece of bone becomes denuded because of stripping of the gingival mucoperiosteum a decision has to be taken regarding the advisability of retaining the bone and risking infection, or removing it with a loss of alveolar support.

As previously noted some injuries to the lower anterior teeth are associated with a 'degloving' laceration of the anterior buccal mucosa. The separation occurs at a supraperiosteal level and in severe cases the mental nerves may be exposed. It is not unusual to find debris or dirt in the depths of the wound and in this situation copious lavage with warm saline is essential. Perhaps surprisingly suture is again rarely necessary and is actually quite difficult because of contusion and friability of the tissues. Healing is normally straightforward although external support strapping will help to adapt the tissues. Prevention of infection is the key to success.

Review and further management

All injured teeth, even following minor trauma, should be reviewed clinically and radiographically to assess the need for further treatment. Root canal therapy will be required in many cases but root resorption may adversely affect the ultimate prognosis. It is important to communicate the details of the injury and emergency treatment carried out to the patient's general dental practitioner, with a reminder to monitor the vitality, colour and clinical condition of the damaged teeth.

Finally, and importantly, it must be recognized that many dental injuries result in medico-legal claims because of the cosmetic and psychological effects of loss of permanent teeth in young adults and the cost of eventual replacement. It is most important that careful clinical records are kept at all stages of treatment.

Further reading

Andreasen JO, Andreasen FM, Andersson L. *Textbook and Colour Atlas of Traumatic Injuries to the Teeth*. Oxford: Wiley-Blackwell; 2007.

Andreasen JO, Baklund LK, Flores MT, Andreasen FM, Andersson L. *Traumatic Dental Injuries: A Manual*. 3rd Edn. Oxford: Wiley-Blackwell; 2011.

Gopikrishna V, Pradeep G, Venkateshbabu N. Assessment of pulp vitality: a review. *Int J Paediatr Dent*. 2009;19:3–15.

Miller SA, Miller G. Use of evidence-based decision-making in private practice for emergency treatment of dental trauma: *J Evid Based Dent Pract*. 2010;10:135–146.

CHAPTER 6

Treatment of fractures of the mandible

Fractures of the mandible are common, yet despite widespread clinical experience and extensive literature on the subject some aspects of care still remain controversial, in particular the management of fractures of the condyle and fractures in severely atrophic jaws. Unfortunately, for a number of reasons, suboptimal outcomes still occur, although traditional complications from infection and malunion are now unusual.

For most fractures of the mandible, the aim of treatment is primarily to restore function, namely to restore both the occlusion and pain-free normal movements of both temporomandibular joints (TMJs). For these goals to be reached, precise anatomical reduction is not essential in every case, although it is clearly desirable. Because of the relatively thick soft tissue coverage of the lower jaw, minor discrepancies in imprecisely anatomically reduced fractures are generally imperceptible in all but the most emaciated of patients.

In undisplaced fractures, 'closed' management simply involves analgesia, judicious use of antibiotics where the fracture is contaminated, and a soft diet until a firm callus has formed. Intermaxillary fixation (IMF) during this time may or may not be required. For displaced or mobile mandibular fractures the general principles of treatment do not differ essentially from the treatment of fractures elsewhere in the body. The fragments are reduced into a good position and are then immobilized until such time as bony union occurs. Traditionally, immobilization of the mandible has involved linking it temporarily to the opposing jaw by some form of IMF. This has the considerable disadvantage to the patient of preventing normal jaw function and restricting the diet to a liquid or semi-solid consistency. Weight loss is common, oral hygiene is difficult to maintain and convalescence is prolonged. In many patients there is also a significant reduction of ventilatory volume.

IMF is also based on the erroneous assumption that if the teeth are placed into occlusion all fractures will automatically be anatomically reduced.

For all these reasons, alternative methods of treatment have been developed that avoid or shorten the period of IMF. The most significant change towards the modern treatment of mandibular fractures, and in particular fractures of the dentate mandible, was the introduction of rigid or semi-rigid osteosynthesis by means of bone plates. The principles of bone healing with rigid or semi-rigid fixation have been outlined in Chapter 1 (p. 7). Transoral semi-rigid fixation by miniature plates (miniplates) is currently the treatment of choice for most mandibular fractures. Rigid 'load-bearing' plate fixation still has a role to play in some complex cases such as extensive comminution, already infected fractures or when concomitant bone grafting is required. Elastic IMF may still be required to 'fine tune' the occlusion where precise anatomical reduction has not been possible but wire IMF, once a mainstay of treatment, is now rarely employed as definitive management.

Consistently successful results from open reduction and internal fixation with miniplates can be expected in most cases. Mandibular fractures are extremely common, however, and in economically less developed countries or in conditions of war access to plating equipment may be limited. The application of mandibular bone plates requires access to operating theatre facilities and special instrumentation, not to mention more advanced training, all of which may not be freely available in all parts of the world. It follows therefore that a considerable proportion of these fractures worldwide will continue to be treated by simpler traditional methods such as the application of IMF and/or wire direct osteosynthesis.

Fractures of the Facial Skeleton, Second Edition. Michael Perry, Andrew Brown and Peter Banks.
© 2015 John Wiley & Sons, Ltd. Published 2015 by John Wiley & Sons, Ltd.

Mandibular fractures in children, fractures of the mandibular condyle and fractures of the edentulous mandible, each present their own particular problems of management that will be considered individually.

Fractures of the tooth-bearing section of the mandible

Reduction

Reduction of a fracture means the restoration of functional alignment of the bone fragments. In certain situations, for example a fracture of the clavicle, this does not necessarily require exact anatomical alignment. However, in the dentate mandible reduction must be precise when healthy occluding teeth are involved. Less precise reduction may be acceptable if the body of the mandible is edentulous or there are no opposing teeth.

The presence of teeth provides a useful guide in most cases by which the related bony fragments can be aligned. This is the principle behind IMF. The teeth are used to assist the reduction, check alignment of the fragments and assist in the immobilization. Whenever the occlusion is used as a guide to fracture reduction it is important to recognize any pre-existing occlusal abnormalities such as an anterior or lateral open bite. Wear facets on individual teeth can provide valuable clues. Teeth may on occasions be brought into contact during reduction and yet be occluding incorrectly owing to lingual inclination of the fracture segment. Widely displaced, multiple or extensively comminuted fractures may be impossible to reduce by means of manipulation of the teeth alone, in which case operative exploration becomes necessary.

In general, reduction and immobilization is best effected under general anaesthesia, but occasionally it is possible to employ local analgesia, supplemented if necessary by sedation. If the patient's general medical condition precludes the administration of a general anaesthetic, gradual reduction of fractures can sometimes be carried out by elastic traction. Small orthodontic elastic bands are applied to modified orthodontic brackets cemented to selected teeth on the individual mandibular fragments and attached in turn to teeth in the intact maxilla. If orthodontic brackets are not available interdental wires or segments of arch bar can be used for the same purpose. A satisfactory

temporary reduction can usually be achieved pending an improvement in the patient's general condition. This immobilization of the fracture also provides pain relief and reduces risks of infection.

Teeth in the fracture line

Teeth in the fracture line are a potential impediment to healing for the following reasons:
1 The fracture is compound into the mouth via the opened periodontal membrane.
2 The tooth may be damaged structurally or lose its blood supply as a result of the trauma so that the pulp subsequently becomes necrotic.
3 The tooth may be affected by some pre-existing pathological process, such as chronic apical infection.

As a result the fracture line may become infected, either from the oral cavity via the disrupted periodontium or directly from an infected pulp or chronic apical granuloma. Infection of the fracture line will result in greatly protracted healing or even non-union.

For these reasons teeth in the line of the fracture were routinely extracted prior to the development of antibiotics. This practice was continued into the antibiotic era with unnecessary detriment to the patient. Generally speaking a tooth in the line of fracture that is structurally undamaged, potentially functional and not subluxed, should be retained and antibiotics administered. Its retention may possibly delay clinical union by a short period, but this is acceptable in order to preserve the integrity of the dentition. Obviously teeth in an intact dentition are more important than those in a partially edentulous jaw.

Without antibiotic therapy teeth in the line of fracture constitute a real risk of infection. However, it is important to remember that other factors are equally important in increasing the risk. It is generally considered that open repair of mandibular fractures should be undertaken as soon as possible. It is often assumed that the longer the delay in repair, the more likely it is that infection will occur. However, what is unclear from the literature is how much of a delay is clinically acceptable. Although some clinicians may feel that a delay of more than a few days may increase the risk studies have failed to demonstrate a direct relationship between delay in repair and increase in complication rates. Excessive fracture mobility, poor oral hygiene and smoking are probably more important in predicting poor outcomes. When prolonged delay is anticipated, temporary support using a 'bridle wire' (a wire loop ligature placed round the necks of teeth adjacent to the fracture) and/or temporary IMF are useful interim measures. In the absence of timely primary management complication rates as high as 30% have been reported. In this situation many publications make the observation that infection is almost invariably associated with teeth in the fracture line but despite this the incidence is not affected by early removal. With the appropriate use of antibiotics and appropriate treatment the infection rate of mandibular fractures that involve teeth is much lower (around 5%). Careful follow-up of any retained teeth is necessary so that endodontic therapy can be immediately instituted where there are clinical indications.

Fractures at the angle of the mandible with teeth in the fracture line appear to be more likely to become infected than at other sites. Controversy therefore exists with regard to the management of functionless third molars involved in a mandibular fracture. These teeth are a potential source of infection and, if left, will eventually probably need to be removed. Furthermore, such a tooth will never be easier to remove because the fracture effectively disimpacts it and as a result it can be elevated with minimal disturbance of bone and periosteum. On balance it would therefore seem sensible to remove a functionless, potentially troublesome tooth when surgical repair is necessary. If a tooth needs to be removed, it is sometimes preferable to pre-plate the fracture first and then remove the plate before elevating the tooth. This is because the tooth itself may help to stabilize the fracture and, once it has been elevated, precise reduction and stabilization of the fracture can become more difficult. Accurate reduction is facilitated by pre-extraction temporary positioning of a fixation plate. Bone removal to allow tooth elevation should always be avoided if possible since it will add to the difficulty in precise alignment.

A summary of the management of any teeth involved in the line of fracture is outlined in Table 6.1.

Immobilization

Following accurate reduction of the fragments, the fracture site must be adequately immobilized to allow bone healing to occur. In orthopaedic practice, uncomplicated repair of the weight-bearing skeleton is of paramount importance in the eventual rehabilitation of an injured patient. As previously discussed, when

Table 6.1 Management of teeth involved in a mandibular fracture line.

a. Absolute indications for removal of a tooth from the fracture line:
  1 Longitudinal fracture involving the root.
  2 Dislocation or subluxation of the tooth from its socket.
  3 Presence of periapical infection.
  4 Advanced periodontal disease.
  5 Already infected fracture line.
  6 Acute pericoronitis.
  7 Where a displaced tooth prevents reduction of the fracture.
b. Relative indications for removal of a tooth from the fracture line:
  1 Functionless tooth that would probably eventually be removed.
  2 Advanced caries.
  3 Doubtful teeth that could be added to existing dentures. (All teeth not covered by these conditions should be retained if possible.)
c. Assessment and treatment of a tooth retained in the fracture line:
  1 Good quality intra-oral periapical radiograph essential.
  2 Institution of appropriate systemic antibiotic therapy.
  3 Splinting of the tooth if mobile.
  4 Endodontic therapy if pulp is exposed.
  5 Immediate extraction if fracture becomes infected.
  6 Follow-up for 1 year and endodontic therapy if there is demonstrable loss of vitality.

semi-rigid fixation is used a fracture heals with the formation of callus. This is a relatively slow process and in a limb weight bearing must be delayed until full bone replacement has occurred. Even apparently 'rigid' fixation using heavier non-compression plates still leaves a gap between the bone ends requiring callus formation. Basically, only compression osteosynthesis results in primary bone healing without the formation of intermediate callus, resulting in more rapid stabilization of the fracture site and much earlier restoration of the mechanical strength of the bone.

These principles have been applied in the treatment of mandibular fractures, but their relevance is questionable. Unlike a weight-bearing bone, it is only necessary to immobilize the mandible until a stable relationship between the fragments has been achieved. This period is considerably less than would be required for full bony consolidation to take place. Some simple mandibular fractures need no immobilization at all, particularly if lack of teeth means that precise restoration of the occlusion is not important. Such fractures may remain mobile for some time if they are tested by careful manipulation but they eventually proceed to full bony union. Indeed it is difficult to prevent a fractured mandible uniting in the absence of infection and malunion is a more frequent complication than non-union.

Infection of a fracture line has traditionally been regarded as a contraindication to any form of direct skeletal fixation. At one time it was considered inadvisable to place any metalwork if the fracture was compound into the mouth because of the risk of subsequent infection. However, with the routine employment of prophylactic antibiotic cover, this risk is considerably reduced. Furthermore, there is now evidence to show that stable plate fixation of previously infected fractures produces better results in terms of uncomplicated healing than traditional closed methods.

The overwhelming advantage of plating techniques is that they are all sufficiently rigid to obviate the need for IMF in most cases. Because clinical union of mandibular fractures is quicker than in most other bones it would seem that compression osteosynthesis offers no significant advantage. One useful role for rigid fixation is to maintain the gross contour of the mandible in the management of comminuted fractures following high impact injuries. For most other fractures, semi-rigid miniplate fixation has proved perfectly adequate in clinical practice.

Period of immobilization

Indirect fixation by the application of IMF is rarely used as the main or only form of immobilization in modern practice. However, if circumstances dictate this form of treatment one thing to be considered is the length of time it will need to be in place to allow stable clinical union to occur. Studies have shown that with early uncomplicated treatment in a healthy young adult union can on average be achieved after 3 weeks, at which time the fixation can be released. As an empirical guide a further 1–2 weeks should be added for each and any of the following circumstances; (1) where a tooth is retained in the fracture line, (2) patients aged 40 years and over, (3) patients who are smokers and (4) mobile or comminuted fractures. Rules such as these are designed for guidance only, and it must be emphasized that the IMF should be released and the fracture tested clinically before the fixation is finally removed.

In most circumstances open reduction and internal plate fixation (ORIF: Open Reduction and Internal Fixation) is now the main form of treatment for mandibular fractures. Although this will generally obviate the need

for IMF the question of how long before union takes place still arises. Return to normal mouth function will depend on uncomplicated wound healing and how quickly the post-operative discomfort settles, both of which will depend on the complexity of the injury. Patients will also vary in their pain perception and the ease of recovery from the surgery and each case has to be considered individually. It is normal practice to advise a soft or even semi-liquid diet for a few weeks but post-operative discomfort, combined with the body's natural protective mechanisms during healing, makes such advice fairly self-evident. All patients who have been treated for a fractured jaw will naturally want to restrict their diet until they feel comfortable to return to a normal eating. In practice this seems to take about 4–6 weeks for all but the toughest foodstuffs. Some patients, such as those involved in contact sports, will want to know when they can return to full physical activity. There is no hard evidence to inform this decision, but once again 6 weeks should be long enough in fit young patients to allow good clinical union to the point where a significant blow would be required to re-fracture the mandible. However, the degree of risk will vary according to the sporting activity and each case must be considered on its merits. Patients should be fully aware that complete bone healing, as opposed to clinical union, will take several months longer.

Methods of immobilization

Fractures of the mandible can be immobilized by various methods of internal direct fixation, the application of IMF or by using external fixation (Table 6.2). On rare occasions a combination of methods may be required.

Direct fixation (osteosynthesis)

This is usually achieved by some form of bone plate, although some oblique fractures can occasionally be fixed by suitably positioned lag screws. Several systems of bone plating are now available for fixation of mandibular fractures and the choice can sometimes be difficult. This is because of the continuing debate over the question of how rigid fixation needs to be in practice. For example, IMF certainly does not rigidly immobilize fractures yet it clearly works and good healing normally takes place. By way of contrast, bone plates based on the Swiss AO/ASIF (Arbeitsgemeinschaft für Osteosynthese/Association for the Study of Internal Fixation) technique are designed to provide

Table 6.2 Methods of immobilization for fractures of the dentate mandibular.

---

a. Direct fixation (Osteosynthesis):
    Semi-rigid plates (miniplates)
    Rigid plates (non-compression)
    Compression plates
    Lag screws
    Resorbable plates and screws
b. IMF:
    Bonded orthodontic brackets
    Inter-dental wiring (direct wiring, eyelet wiring etc.)
    Arch bars
    IMF Screws
c. External fixation
d. Other methods (largely historical or where plates not available):
    Transosseous wiring
    Circumferential wiring
    Transfixion (Kirschner wires)

---

complete rigidity across the fracture, sometimes with a degree of compression.

In clinical use each plating system, rigid or semi-rigid, normally ensures sufficient strength of fixation across the fracture site to obviate the need for IMF. This enables the patient to continue to enjoy a relatively soft diet and to maintain oral hygiene more easily. These conditions are clearly desirable for all mandibular fractures but in certain cases they are highly desirable. For example, a fracture of the body of the mandible with a coexistent intracapsular fracture of the condyle may make early mobilization especially important in order to ensure recovery of function of the temporomandibular joint. IMF is not well tolerated in some very young or elderly patients and is particularly difficult to maintain in mentally agitated patients or those with severe learning difficulties.

However, the application of bone plates to the mandible is an exacting technique requiring general anaesthesia in most cases and a considerable degree of surgical skill. Specialized instrumentation is usually needed to facilitate the desired intra-oral approach. Occasionally an extra-oral approach will be needed, for example in grossly comminuted fractures.

Any treatment method that does not rely on IMF must ensure the precise restoration of the occlusion. Even though bone plates are placed with the benefit of visual open reduction they do not always achieve this fundamental objective because true anatomical repositioning can be quite difficult in some fractures. ORIF is an unforgiving technique and some series have shown that up to 25% of treated cases may require a degree of occlusal adjustment post-operatively. To minimize this problem many operators still advise a short period of IMF, particularly in more complex cases.

The reported incidence of postoperative infection of bone plates seems to be decreasing and plating may indeed be employed for the elective treatment of infected fractures. Some of these improved results can be attributed to greater surgical skill, antibiotics and the use of more biocompatible materials. Titanium has now replaced stainless steel and chrome-cobalt alloys for the manufacture of all types of plates. Although there may be theoretical reasons for removal of metal plates on the grounds that they protect the underlying bone from normal stress and therefore may lead to atrophic changes, there is still no convincing evidence to indicate the need for them to be removed routinely. Most surgeons leave asymptomatic plates *in situ*. A few plates may have to be removed due to infection and in some centres routine elective removal is the norm. Older materials may cause artefacts on CT scans and possible difficulties with MRI scans, but this is not a significant problem with titanium.

However, to complicate the issue, there is now some evidence that titanium is not quite as biologically inert as was originally supposed. Limited corrosion takes place with detectable particles in both local tissue and regional lymph nodes. These findings have reinforced the argument made by some for the routine removal of all metal plates. Of course this raises the question that, if all plates are going to be removed why use a more expensive material like titanium in the first place rather than stainless steel?

For all of these various reasons maxillofacial surgeons as well as orthopaedic surgeons have looked for a biodegradable material that could be used in the construction of sufficiently strong bone plates. The most obvious available biocompatible and absorbable material is bone itself, either autogenous or bank bone. Interestingly there are records of individual patients from World War I that describe the use of screws and dowels fashioned from bone used to fix mandibular fractures and bone grafts in an effort to avoid the ever present risk of infection.

Research on resorbable plates has concentrated on a group of high molecular weight poly-alpha-hydroxy acids and their copolymers. Commercially produced plating systems generally use copolymers of laevo and dextro lactic acid in various proportions, which are formed into small plates that are heat malleable, resorbed within two years and strong enough for craniofacial reconstruction. One disadvantage is the need for careful tapping of the screw holes, and the screws and plates are bulkier than their equivalent metal counterparts. A number of studies and reviews have compared titanium plates to resorbable when used in mandibular fractures and orthognathic surgery. In general equal results are obtained, but despite this resorbable plates have not been widely adopted. The reason seems to be that in the final analysis they are technically more time consuming to apply and no clear advantage over metal plate fixation has so far been demonstrated.

Semi-rigid plates (miniplates)

These are the commonest form of internal fixation used in the management of mandibular fractures. The earliest types of small mandibular plates were based on chrome-cobalt orthopaedic metacarpal plates and were not widely accepted. However, plating techniques rapidly gained in popularity with the development in the 1970s by Michelet and Champy of customized miniature plates and sets of instruments designed specifically for maxillofacial use. They were originally fabricated in stainless steel but titanium is now the metal of choice, with a large variety of plates of various designs widely available and in routine use (Fig. 6.1).

The original developers of mandibular miniplates argued that compression plates were unnecessary because there was a natural line of compression along the lower border of the mandible. They further argued that rigid and compression plates exerted a stress shielding effect that was detrimental to ultimate mandibular strength. Non-compression miniplates with screw fixation confined to the outer cortex allow the operator more freedom in siting the plates both sub-apically as well as in the region of the lower border. On the basis of experimental studies using stressed mandibular models it has been shown that fractures at the angle can be secured with a single plate as near to the upper border as the anatomy permits (Fig. 6.2a). Tension forces in this region are then converted to compressive forces along the entire fracture (a concept known as 'load sharing' osteosynthesis). A plate placed at the angle region is

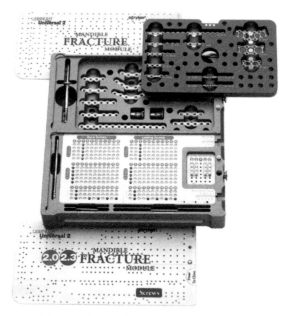

Figure 6.1 Typical example of different shapes and sizes of plates available for the fixation of fractures of the facial skeleton. (Reproduced with kind permission of Springer Science+Business Media.)

shaped to lie along the external oblique ridge, or can be placed more laterally on the flatter aspect of the mandible by using a trans-buccal trochar and cannula to place the screws. In the canine and symphyseal region two plates at least 5 mm apart are required to resist the torsional effects of the anterior mandibular musculature. One is placed in the juxta-alveolar region and one towards the lower border. Care needs to be taken when fixing plates close to the mental foramen (Fig. 6.2b). Protection of the mental nerve whilst drilling the holes and inserting the screws is paramount. All plates can be inserted by an intra-oral approach without the routine need for additional IMF.

Open reduction and internal fixation (ORIF) of mandibular fractures is now the accepted method of treatment in most maxillofacial centres, although traditional methods of indirect fixation will still have a place where access to plating equipment is limited. As mentioned previously, ORIF is technique sensitive and most published series report a small incidence of minor residual malocclusion requiring post-operative adjustment. Similarly, a number of patients will require plate removal due to infection. Despite these reported problems the advantages of direct fixation without the

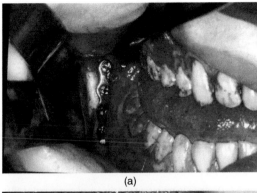

(a)

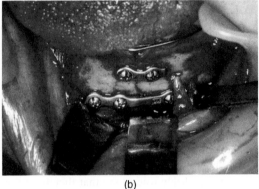

(b)

Figure 6.2 Open reduction and internal fixation (ORIF) of a bilateral fracture of the mandible using an intraoral approach and titanium miniplates with monocortical screws. (a) Fracture of right angle fixed with a single plate adapted to lie along the upper border and external oblique ridge. (b) Left parasymphyseal fracture. In this area two plates are needed to achieve stable fixation. A temporary 'bridle wire' is visible in the upper part of the picture. This was placed around a number of firm teeth either side of the fracture in order to stabilize the reduction during application of the plates.

need for IMF far outweigh any disadvantages and have proved convincing in practice.

Miniplate osteosynthesis can be used in most common types of mandibular fracture, with plates inserted via an intra-oral approach. It is only necessary to reflect periosteum from the outer plate of bone. This is an advantage when compared with the older methods of transosseous wiring. The plates are pre-bent to lay passively across the fracture line with a minimum of two, and preferably three, screw holes available either side. Mono-cortical fixation with 2.0 mm screws is performed. Straightforward fractures can be reduced and plated whilst an assistant supports the mandible in a firmly closed position against the intact maxilla.

Difficult to reduce fractures in the anterior region can be stabilized by using a 'bridle wire' (Fig. 6.2b) or inserting a screw either side of the fracture and placing a temporary 'tie-wire' to approximate the bone ends whilst the plates are inserted. However, comminuted or mobile fractures may ultimately be difficult to reduce and stabilize without the use of temporary intra-operative IMF. Some surgeons advise this as routine when placing miniplates in order to minimize the risk of postoperative occlusal discrepancies. For the same reason a short period of post-operative elastic IMF may be advised in difficult or complex fractures.

As mentioned above, the plates can usually be left in place permanently without causing trouble. Similarly, although there is now firm evidence that corrosion and local dispersal of titanium does take place this is only detectable by ultra-microscopic techniques and, while this is quoted by some as another reason for routine plate removal, its significance long-term has yet to be evaluated.

Non-compression rigid plates

Several types of larger profile plates (e.g. 2.3–2.7 mm) are now available that can provide near rigid, or 'load bearing', osteosynthesis. These are not used for routine fracture management by most surgeons but definitely have a place in the management of infected or severely comminuted fractures (Fig. 6.3). They are also useful in fractures where there are continuity defects, and in fractures in which delayed union or non-union has occurred. The key to success in managing these types of fractures is to immobilize them sufficiently to allow enough vascularization for healing to occur. Adaptation of the plates is obviously technically more demanding and, since they are usually longer than miniplates, they often require an extra-oral approach for accurate placement.

Rigid plates require bicortical screws and are fixed in place at or near the lower border of the mandible in order to avoid damage to the inferior alveolar nerve and the dental roots. At least three screws are inserted either side of the fracture and care is taken to ensure that all screws are perpendicular to the bone surface. Some modern designs of plates employ locking screws that lock into the plate at the completion of insertion in order to avoid any micro-movement between the plate and the screw. This is thought to minimize any tendency to loosening of the fixation and plate failure.

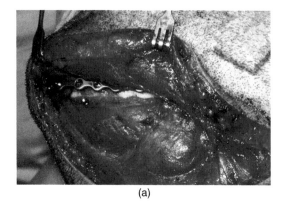

(a)

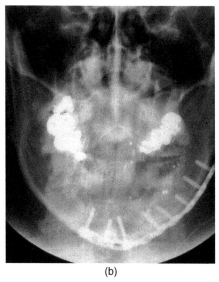

(b)

Figure 6.3 (a) Extra-oral approach used to treat a comminuted fracture of left mandible caused by a blow from a baseball bat. A rigid non-compression plate has been placed at the lower border. The head of a single lag screw inserted from the lower border across an oblique fracture can also be seen. (b) PA radiograph of reduced fracture with plate *in situ*.

The use of rigid plates raises concerns about stress shielding of the underlying bone that reduces functional load bearing adaptation in the longer term and removal is often advised for this reason. In addition they may become palpable beneath the skin and removal may be requested by the patient.

Compression plates
The theory and practice behind compression osteosynthesis of mandibular fractures is based on the similar treatment of fractures of weight bearing long bones

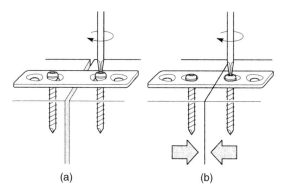

(a)   (b)

Figure 6.4 Diagram to represent the theory of compression plating. During final tightening of the screw head in the eccentric pear-shaped hole (a) there is inward movement as it slides into the wider part and (b) thus pushes the bone fragments together.

(Fig. 6.4). However, as has been previously pointed out, non-union or delayed union is rarely a problem in fractures of the mandible or other facial bones. In addition precise reduction is essential in the dentate mandible. This is difficult to achieve when using compression plating techniques and, for these and other reasons, it is probably true to say that they have now been abandoned by the majority of maxillofacial units. For the interested reader it may be instructive to explain further why this has occurred.

As for all rigid plates, compression plates are secured to the convex outer surface of the mandible surface using bicortical screws and they must therefore be sited below the inferior alveolar canal. However skilfully the plate is adapted, there is still a tendency for both the upper border and the lingual plate to open with the tightening of the compression screws. This leads both to distortion of the occlusion and, in a bilateral fracture, to opening of the fracture line on the other side.

Because of this tendency for the upper border to open when compression is applied across the fracture, it is necessary to apply a so-called 'tension band' at the dentoalveolar level before tightening the screws. This can be in the form of an arch bar ligated to the teeth or as a separate plate with screws penetrating the outer cortex only (Fig. 6.5). The operative approach for compression plates tends to be lengthy and requires considerable expertise to produce consistent results. Over time it has become increasingly apparent that they offer no material advantage to the patient in the treatment of facial bone fractures.

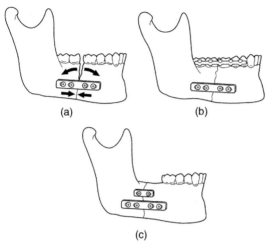

(a)   (b)

(c)

Figure 6.5 Diagram illustrating the major problem with compression plating of the mandible. (a) A single plate near the lower border tends to open up the fracture at the alveolar level unless a 'tension band' is also placed; either (b) an arch bar or (c) a second smaller plate.

Lag screws

A few oblique fractures of the mandible can be rigidly immobilized by inserting two or more screws whose threads engage only the inner plate of bone. The hole drilled in the outer cortex is made to a slightly larger diameter than the threaded part of the screw. When tightened the head of the screw therefore impinges on the outer plate and the oblique fracture is compressed (Fig. 6.6). At least two such lag screws are necessary to achieve rigid immobilization.

Resorbable plates and screws

As has been discussed previously, the theoretical advantages of using bioabsorbable plates and screws have not proved to be conclusive in actual clinical practice. The materials used have a somewhat lengthy period of degradation that may not end in total absorption, although this does not appear to be a problem clinically. The main criticism has been a failure to demonstrate a convincing advantage over the more popular and easier to use titanium plates. Apart from an accepted place in paediatric craniofacial surgery resorbable plates have few advocates for routine use in facial trauma.

Intermaxillary fixation (IMF)

In the presence of sufficient numbers of teeth, simple fractures of the tooth-bearing part of the mandible may

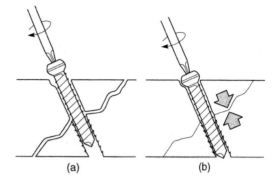

(a)   (b)

Figure 6.6 Diagram to illustrate the principle of lag screws. The thread only engages the deeper section of bone (a) and thus compression is applied as the screw is tightened (b).

be adequately immobilized by IMF alone. This was, of course, the conventional method of treatment prior to the development of effective plating techniques. Clinical union can be expected within 4 weeks in nearly all cases and the fixation can often be established without resorting to general anaesthesia. Today, IMF is most frequently used as a temporary measure to maintain the correct occlusion while some form of direct osteosynthesis is applied. In some complex cases a short period of IMF, often using 'guiding' elastics, may be needed to supplement direct fixation. A number of methods of IMF are available, most of which have a long history of clinical use in maxillofacial surgery.

Bonded orthodontic brackets

Fractures with minimal displacement in patients with good oral hygiene can be immobilized by bonding a number of modified orthodontic brackets, or short segments of arch bar, onto the teeth and applying light wires or intermaxillary elastic bands (Fig. 6.7). If access to a maxillofacial laboratory is available orthodontic brackets can be suitably prepared by welding small hooks onto each of them. Selected teeth in each jaw are carefully dried, etched and the brackets bonded to them with composite resin. Because this technique depends on as dry an environment as possible it is difficult to use in cases where there is anything other than minimal intra-oral bleeding. This method may be particularly useful for treating fractures in younger patients.

Inter-dental wiring

Inter-dental wiring is only applicable when the patient has a complete, or almost complete, number of suitably

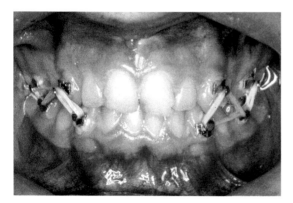

Figure 6.7 Immobilization of a fractured mandible in a young patent by bonding small brackets onto teeth and applying inter-maxillary fixation with orthodontic elastics.

shaped teeth. Opinions differ as to the type and gauge of wire used, but 0.45 mm soft stainless wire has been found to be effective. This wire requires stretching before use by about 10%. If this is not done the wires become slack after being in position a few days. Care should be taken not to over-stretch the wire as it will become work hardened and brittle. Numerous techniques have been described for inter-dental wiring, but the two simple methods described next have been found satisfactory in most instances.

Direct wiring. This is the simplest method. The middle portion of a 15 cm (6 inch) length of wire is twisted round a suitable tooth and then the free ends are twisted together to produce a 7.5–10 cm (3–4 inch) length of 'plaited' wire. Similar wires are attached to other teeth elsewhere in the upper and lower jaws and then after reduction of the fracture the plaited ends of wires in the upper and lower jaws are in turn twisted together. For greater stability the wire surrounding each tooth can be applied in the form of a clove hitch. Thus suitable teeth in the upper and lower jaws are joined together by direct wires.

This is a simple method of immobilizing the jaws, which can provide rapid temporary IMF during the application of direct fixation. The disadvantage as a longer form of fixation arises from the fact that the intermaxillary wires are connected to the teeth themselves. It is therefore difficult to release the intermaxillary connection without stripping off the entire fixation. This disadvantage is overcome by using interdental eyelet wiring or similar techniques.

Eyelet wiring. Eyelets are constructed by holding a 15 cm (6 inch) length of wire by a pair of artery forceps at either end and giving the middle of the wire two turns around a piece of round bar of 3 mm (1/8 inch) diameter, such as the shaft of a long surgical bur, which is fixed securely in a clamp or vice.

Eyelets are fitted around a pair of teeth and twisted tight as shown in Fig. 6.8. Care must be taken to push the wire well down on the lingual and palatal aspect of the teeth before twisting the free ends tight or the eyelet will tend to 'ride up' coronally and become loose.

Four to six eyelets should be so positioned in both the upper and the lower jaw that when the tie wires are threaded through them a cross-bracing effect is achieved. If the eyelets are placed immediately above each other some mobility of the mandible will usually still be possible. It should be remembered when working with wire that precautions must be taken to protect the patient's eyes at all times. Every free end of wire should be prevented from accidentally damaging tissues by having a pair of heavy artery forceps attached to it when it is not actually being manipulated.

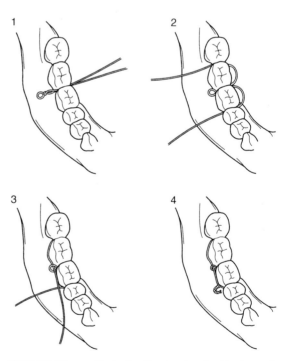

Figure 6.8 Diagram illustrating the steps involved in the application of an eyelet wire.

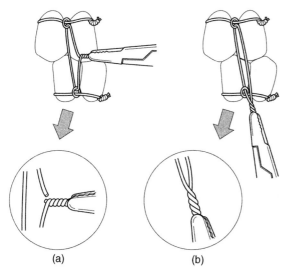

Figure 6.9 Incorrect (a) and correct (b) method of tightening intermaxillary tie wires. Breakage is common if the wire is held in the forceps at right angles to the loop as it is pulled and twisted tightly. It is better to position the twisted portion close to an eyelet as shown to minimize sharp angulation of the wire.

After the eyelet wires have been applied the tie wires should be loosely threaded through the eyelets in the opposing jaws. Any throat packing is removed, after which the fracture is reduced by bringing the jaws together and the tie wire fixation is tightened (Fig. 6.9).

It is important that the patient's normal pre-fracture occlusion is fully appreciated by the surgeon, particularly when working under general anaesthesia when muscle relaxation is present. Many patients have some abnormality of their occlusion and a mistaken attempt to achieve a theoretically correct position in such cases may result in misalignment of the bony fragments, a fact that may not be immediately obvious during closed reduction. Information about the previous occlusion can often be inferred from wear facets on the teeth.

In order to re-establish the occlusion and avoid a cross-bite, the tie wires should initially be tightened in the molar area, first on one side and then on the other, working round to the incisor teeth. Wires may be twisted quite tightly on multi-rooted teeth, but some caution should be exercised with single-rooted teeth to avoid subluxation. It is best to twist the tie wires loosely together first and carry out the definitive tightening only after the occlusion has finally been checked. Care must be taken to ensure that the tongue is not trapped

between the cusps of the teeth. After the interdental eyelet wiring is completed a finger should be run round the patient's mouth to ensure that no loose ends of wire have been left projecting that may ulcerate the soft tissue.

Interdental eyelet wiring is simple to apply and very effective in practice. If facilities for ORIF are not available a majority of dentate mandibular fractures can still be treated in this fashion. To test whether a fracture is soundly united is simply a matter of removing the tie wires. If a further period of immobilization is indicated new tie wires can be attached.

Eyelet wires can be modified to allow the use of elastic IMF if required (Fig. 6.10) and many other adaptations of interdental wiring techniques have been described in the literature.

Arch bars

Arch bars are perhaps the most versatile form of IMF. They are often used for the application of temporary or light elastic IMF ('guiding elastics') to supplement ORIF when required. If IMF is employed as the definitive method of treatment for a fracture then arch bars are indicated where the patient has an insufficient number of suitably shaped teeth to enable effective interdental eyelet wiring to be carried out or when, in an otherwise intact arch, a direct linkage across the fracture is required.

The method is very simple. The fracture is reduced and the teeth on the main fragments are individually

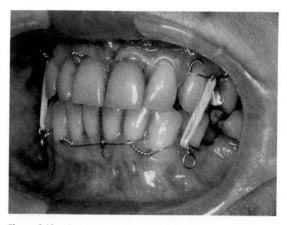

Figure 6.10 Elastic 'guiding' IMF applied using modified eyelet wires. A few extra twists to the eyelet portion increases the length allowing them to be bent as a hook for the elastic band.

ligated to a bar that has been shaped to conform to the dental arch. Many varieties of prefabricated arch bar are commercially available that have suitable hooks for the attachment of intermaxillary elastic or wire fixation. A simpler alternative, such as notched 3 mm half-round German silver bar, will sometimes suffice if IMF wires rather than elastics are indicated (Fig. 6.11). Arch bars should be cut to the required length and bent to the correct shape before starting the operation. If the mandibular fragments are displaced the bar can be shaped initially using the intact upper arch as a guide. In practice direct application to the lower arch is usually quite straightforward as extreme accuracy is not essential.

It is helpful after the arch bar has been formed to commence wiring on adjacent teeth, preferably in the midline. The arch bar is wired to successive teeth on each side working backwards to each third molar area.

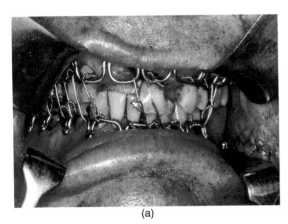

(a)

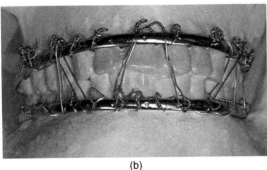

(b)

Figure 6.11 (a) Mandibular fracture treated with IMF using Jelenko pattern arch bars ligated to upper and lower teeth. (b) Models demonstrating the use of simple half-round arch bars. Small notches cut into the bars will prevent lateral slippage of the IMF wires. (Reproduced with kind permission of Springer Science+Business Media.)

In this way minor discrepancies in the arch bar are 'ironed out' as wiring proceeds, producing close adaptation of the bar to the dental arch. Short, approximately 15 cm (6 inch), lengths of either 0.45 mm or 0.35 mm wire are used for each ligature. Each wire is passed over the bar, around the tooth, and then under the bar before the ends are twisted together. Whenever contact points between the teeth are tight, 0.35 mm wire is used. After all the wires have been placed it will inevitably be found that some have become loose and it is therefore important to re-tighten each wire before the twisted portion is cut and tucked into a position where it will not irritate the tissues.

Arch bars are usually placed to allow the application of light IMF elastics as a support for transosseous fixation but, as with inter-dental wiring, they can be used with wire or strong elastic IMF for definitive treatment. Most fractures of the mandible can be effectively treated in this fashion if teeth are present on the main fragments. Occasionally some minimally displaced anterior fractures can be managed with a lower arch bar alone but case selection is extremely important. In this situation the lower teeth and arch bar essentially act like a miniature external fixator.

IMF screws

True inter-*maxillary* fixation can be achieved by anchoring the method used direct to the bone rather than the teeth. Techniques for this purpose include circum-mandibular and piriform fossa wires, or custom made bone hooks that engage with the lower border of the mandible and the piriform fossa. Both these techniques have now largely been superseded by the easier and quicker method of inserting IMF screws. These are particularly useful for the rapid application of intra-operative IMF, which is a helpful aid to stabilizing reduced fractures whilst they are plated.

Custom designed bicortical screws that are both self-drilling and self-tapping are available in variable lengths. For short periods of intra-operative IMF a suitable long screw from the plating set being used will often suffice. The screws are placed directly through the free mucosa, or if preferred through a small 'stab' incision, and inter-maxillary wire ligatures are tied around the slightly protruding screw heads. Care is required in screw placement if there are any teeth nearby and it is obvious that an adequate number of opposing teeth are still required in order for the occlusion to be stable

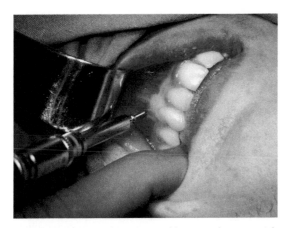

Figure 6.12 IMF screw being inserted between the upper right canine and first premolar. Care is needed to avoid damage to the adjacent roots. If IMF screws are simply to be used for intraoperative stabilization they can sometimes be placed in the safer area beyond the apical region. However, difficulty of subsequent access and problems with ulceration preclude this location for longer term use. (Reproduced with kind permission of Springer Science+Business Media.)

while held in IMF. This is a very rapid way of applying IMF. Each screw is secured to the dentoalveolar bone by inserting it carefully in the interdental space between the roots of the adjacent teeth, or beyond the apical region if this is feasible (Fig. 6.12). Both buccal and lingual/palatal cortices of the bone should be engaged for the screw to remain secure. Because it is essentially a 'blind' procedure suitable radiographs of the jaws are advised beforehand to check root morphology of the adjacent teeth and, particularly in younger patients, to make sure there are no unerupted teeth.

External fixation

With the development of newer, stronger and more biocompatible materials used for internal fixation many of the traditional indications for external fixation no longer apply. Infected fractures were once an absolute contraindication to internal fixation but it is now understood that it is a combination of movement and infection that predisposes to the development of osteomyelitis. If rigidity can be achieved by effective internal fixation then the vascularity of the infected site will improve and the fracture will normally heal. Continuity defects and comminuted fractures once managed by external fixation can now usually be stabilized by internal rigid bridging plates or a series of smaller internal fixation plates.

Nevertheless, external fixation may still have a role in a few selected cases, particularly in pathological fractures due to intra-bony disease or for rapid stabilization of missile injuries prior to transfer. Traditionally a simple set of threaded bone pins, rods and universal joints were used but a number of custom made external fixators are now available. The principle of external fixation is very simple. Ideally, at least two self-tapping screw pins are placed either side of the fracture or defect. The fracture is then reduced and the pins linked by an external bar framework. This type of pin fixation is not absolutely rigid and supplementary IMF is often required. A simple fixation bar can also be fabricated by injecting self-curing acrylic resin into an endotracheal tube (Fig. 6.13).

Historically, this type of fixation has been advocated for the definitive management of missile injuries of the mandible, but currently the main role for external

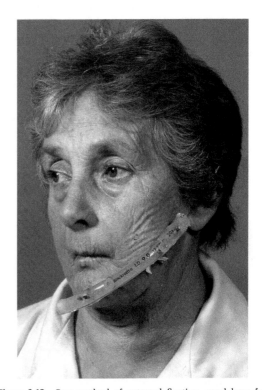

Figure 6.13 One method of external fixation, used here for an infected fracture of the left mandible. Two screw pins have been inserted into each fragment and a length of endotracheal tube pushed over the protruding ends prior to the injection of self-curing acrylic resin. External fixation is rarely indicated and has been superseded in most situations by internal fixation techniques.

fixation in the conflict arena is to provide rapid 'first aid' stabilization of very mobile fractures in the multiply injured patient prior to transfer to a definitive care centre. In addition, external fixation can be used for extended intermediate fixation of contaminated injuries and is useful for maintaining space and orientation in continuity defects.

The main indications for the use of pin fixation for mandibular fractures may therefore be summarized as follows:

1 To provide fixation across an infected fracture line.
2 To stabilize a pathological fracture or where there is a large amount of bone loss.
3 To maintain the relative position of major fragments in extensively comminuted fractures.

Other methods of fixation

A perusal of the extensive literature on the treatment of mandibular fractures will soon reveal that numerous other methods of fixation and immobilization have been described. In the economically advantaged world most of these are now mainly of historical interest, including transosseous upper and lower border bone wiring (Fig. 6.14), circum-mandibular wiring and Kirschner wire transfixion. The advent of ORIF plating techniques has made obsolete many of these previously common methods of treatment in most situations. Despite this, there may still be clinical circumstances in some parts of the world where a resourceful surgeon will need to be able to call upon them.

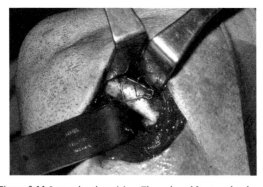

Figure 6.14 Lower border wiring. The reduced fracture has been stabilized by a direct interosseous wire and a separate 'figure of eight' wire around the lower border. Although this technique has been superseded by the use of plates and has the added disadvantage of requiring an external approach it can still achieve excellent fixation. It may occasionally have a place in situations where plating equipment is not readily available.

Fractures of the tooth bearing section of the mandible: synopsis

1 Accurate reduction is essential if there is a good functional occlusion.
2 All of these fractures are compound into the mouth.
3 Teeth in the line of fracture are a potential source of infection and delayed healing.
4 The mandible can be immobilized by direct osteosynthesis, IMF or a combination of both.
5 Non-compression miniplate fixation is currently the preferred method wherever the necessary resources are available.
6 Although compression plating is based on sound general orthopaedic principles these are less relevant to the treatment of mandibular fractures than to the skeleton as a whole.
7 Malunion is much more likely than non-union.

Fractures of the mandible in children

Fractures of the mandible are uncommon in children owing to the fact that young bone is resilient and considerable force is required to effect a fracture. Approximately 8–15% of jaw fractures occur in children under the age of 15 years and only 1% of mandibular fractures happen before the age of 6 years. Some modifications to the foregoing principles of treatment are necessary when the fracture occurs in a child. The line of demarcation between the medulla and cortex is less well defined than in adults and the ratio of tooth to bone substance is high. Incomplete disjunction in the form of a 'greenstick' fracture is therefore more likely and there is a greater risk of damage to developing teeth than in later years. In one long-term investigation of mandibular fractures occurring before the age of 12 years there was developmental disturbance in approximately 70% of teeth directly in the line of fracture.

The treatment of mandibular fractures in children before puberty is generally of a conservative nature because of the rapidity of healing and the adaptive potential of the bone and its contained dentition. However, there are a few special factors that need to be taken into account in managing these injuries.

Interference with growth potential

The normal growth of the mandible will be disturbed if unerupted permanent teeth or teeth germs are lost. This is because the alveolus will not develop normally in the areas affected. Damage to the growth potential will be more severe in the event of infection of the fracture site. One careful cephalometric analysis of 28 children who had experienced mandibular fractures at sites other than the condyle found the mandibular unit length to be less than expected in 67%. One-third of the patients with fractures in the tooth-bearing portion of the mandible had specific dental complications.

The capacity for preferential growth in the sub-condylar region may be seriously compromised by high condylar fractures, particularly if function is restricted as a result of fibrous or bony ankylosis of the temporomandibular joint. The treatment of these injuries is discussed in more detail below.

Fixation in the deciduous and mixed dentition period

In the relatively uncommon situation where the severity and displacement of the fracture are of sufficient degree to warrant immobilization of the mandible, some modification of technique is required. This is because of the presence of unerupted or partially erupted permanent teeth and deciduous teeth of variable mobility.

Fixation independent of the teeth

A simple elasticated bandage chin support may be used in cases with minimal displacement where jaw movement is nevertheless painful.

In the very young with unerupted or very few deciduous teeth a Gunning-type splint for the lower jaw alone may be used. This is constructed as a simple acrylic trough that is soft lined and retained by two light circumferential wires.

Very rarely, when there is significant displacement of fragments, open reduction may be necessary. In this situation any plate or wire fixation must be strictly confined to the lower border to avoid damage to developing teeth (see the following).

Fixation utilizing the teeth

Because open reduction is often contra-indicated due to the risk of damage to the developing dentition orthodontic brackets bonded directly to erupted teeth may be the best way to immobilize the fracture (see Fig. 6.7). Alternatively, where there are sufficient firm erupted deciduous and permanent teeth, eyelet wires or arch bars can be used. It is often difficult to fix wires firmly to deciduous molars and canines but this

may be possible using thinner more flexible soft stainless steel wires of 0.35 mm diameter. Similarly, a light arch bar without hooks is more easily adapted to the irregular mixed dentition and this should be attached to the teeth by similar 0.35 mm diameter wire ligatures.

Simple fractures can sometimes be managed without IMF by cementing a vacuum formed splint over the teeth, supported by circum-mandibular wires if necessary. This type of splint is also useful for paediatric dentoalveolar fractures (see Fig. 5.6, p. 66).

The presence of unerupted teeth

In patients below the age of 9 or 10 years the body of the mandible is congested with developing teeth. As already mentioned, in these circumstances it is unsafe to insert bone plates or transosseous wires. In exceptional instances such as gross displacement of a symphysis or angle fracture a small miniplate may be applied with the shortest possible screws to the lower border, or a transosseous wire inserted with caution.

Healing and remodelling

Mandibular fractures in young children heal very rapidly and some fractures are stable within a week, and firmly united within 3 weeks. If the fragments are firm, but not perfectly reduced, it is as well to accept some slight imperfection in the reduction rather than re-fracture the mandible with possible damage to developing teeth. Similarly, some imperfection in reduction can be accepted when a fresh fracture is treated, as in each of the previous circumstances continuing growth and eruption of teeth will compensate in most cases for the imperfect alignment the fragments.

Prolonged follow-up is required following most fractures of the mandible in children in order to be sure that there are no long-term effects on both mandibular growth and the normal development of the permanent dentition. There are often damaged teeth associated with fractures in this age group and close cooperation with the paedodontist, orthodontist and the patient's general dental practitioner is of vital importance.

Fractures of the mandible in children: synopsis

1 Modification of the principles of treatment is necessary to take account of:
   a. capacity for rapid bony union – fractures are stable between 1 and 3 weeks;

b. the mixed dentition and multiple buried developing teeth;

c. potential interference with subsequent growth.

2 Accurate reduction is less important as further growth
will often compensate for occlusal discrepancies.

3 Direct osteosynthesis should be avoided if possible.
However, plating or wiring the lower border may
occasionally be indicated.

4 IMF can be applied to deciduous teeth if needed
but finer diameter wire should be used. Bonded
orthodontic brackets are preferred if possible.

5 Fractures of the condyle require special consideration.

6 A prolonged period of follow-up is important.

Fractures of the condylar region

Fractures involving the mandibular condyle are the only
facial bone fractures that involve a synovial joint. Injury
to the joint can occur in the absence of any fracture of
the articular surfaces. Trauma to this region may therefore be divided into three main types:

1 *Contusion*: apart from damage to the capsular ligaments, such an injury may be accompanied by a
synovial effusion, haemarthrosis or tearing of the
meniscus. Such injuries are difficult to diagnose
without special imaging techniques but they may
predispose to later degenerative changes in some
cases.

2 *Traumatic dislocation*: irreducible displacement of the
condyle from the glenoid fossa is usually anterior
and/or medial. Lateral, posterior or central dislocations rarely occur. A coexisting fracture of the
condylar neck is common.

3 *Fracture*: includes any fracture above the level of the
sigmoid notch. Fractures, fracture/dislocations and
dislocations of the condyle are all accompanied by
varying degrees of contusion. If the fracture extends
into the joint space, haemarthrosis and rupture of the
meniscus is more likely to occur and such injuries
may predispose to later disturbance of function.

The incidence of condylar fractures as a proportion of
all fractures of the mandible is high and almost 50% of
condylar fractures are associated with other coexistent
fractures of the mandible.

Unfortunately, despite much recent interest in open
reduction techniques, there are still no definitive guidelines for the treatment of fractures of the mandibular

condyle and this remains a controversial topic. One
possible definition of a successful outcome from treatment of a condylar fracture is when the patient can
open his/her mouth fully without deviation of the chin
and can masticate easily with the contralateral side of
the dentition, which implies the recovery of condylar
excursion. These are the criteria for complete functional
recovery. However, clinical experience suggests that
many 'successfully' treated cases fall short of this ideal
if carefully examined.

Conservative management of condylar fractures

Although there are vociferous advocates for open reduction and fixation of most displaced condylar fractures
many authorities continue to argue that this is in practice
rarely necessary. In those patients in whom the fracture
is minimally displaced and the occlusion is undisturbed,
management can be nonsurgical with the prescription
of rest, soft diet and simple analgesics. Regular review is
essential in the early stages of healing to ensure that the
fracture does not 'slip' and heal in an incorrect position.

Unilateral fractures that are significantly displaced and
associated with a malocclusion will need to be actively
treated, but not all need to be anatomically reduced and
plated. The questions then remain:

1 Which fractures should be openly reduced and
repaired surgically?

2 Which fractures should be repaired surgically as
a result of the radiographic findings? Namely,
should treatment be based on the type of fracture
displacement even if the occlusion is essentially
undisturbed?

The traditional approach to the management of
displaced fractures that are not repaired surgically has
been initially to apply IMF. Although wire fixation
can be applied this is more usually carried out with
arch bars and elastic IMF that encourages a functional
realignment of the fragments. The fixation is usually
applied for no more than 10–21 days since it has been
suggested that prolonged IMF can result in capsular
contraction and limitation of mouth opening. However,
there is no strong evidence for this, particularly if
active mobilization is encouraged with the help of
physiotherapy if necessary.

Historically, the majority of surgeons favoured this
conservative approach, avoiding direct disturbance of
the fracture site and concentrating on early restoration

of function. However, a good early functional result does not necessarily mean full recovery of condylar excursion and there is some evidence that subsequent joint dysfunction and osteoarthritis can still occur.

Prospective studies have revealed a number of interesting observations. In the majority of young patients, following fracture of the condyle with displacement, there is a complete anatomical restitution of the temporomandibular articulation within a two-year period. However, in teenagers the joint does not return to normality to the same extent and in adults only minor remodelling is observed. Asymmetry of mandibular movement and altered function at the fracture site usually disappears in children while it persists or becomes aggravated in adults. Late symptoms such as clicking and tenderness are rare in children and frequent amongst adults. These studies suggest that remodelling following displaced fractures can be expected to be anatomical or 'restitutional' in children, and adjusting or 'functional' in adults.

Similarly, another long-term follow-up study in children concluded that the older the child at the time of injury the less the capacity for functional remodelling, due to reduced bone resorptive capacity. Frequent joint dysfunction was noted in these, by now, young adults but in none was this considered serious. Only half of these patients showed complete anatomical restitutional remodelling but the functional result appeared satisfactory in all cases.

Finally, it has been suggested that many cases of osteoarthritis or recurrent dislocation of the TMJ are linked to previous trauma, and that over 60% of cases of ankylosis are associated with previous injury in childhood.

Open reduction of condylar fractures

Grossly displaced fracture dislocations of the condyle, particularly bilateral fractures, are inevitably accompanied by some degree of malocclusion in the dentate patient. Simple immobilization of the mandible by means of wire or elastic IMF does not usually achieve a satisfactory reduction of the fracture and malocclusion persists after healing is complete. Functional distraction of the condyle by applying IMF with the bite propped open posteriorly has been recommended in the past but this is also not a reliable method. ORIF of displaced condylar neck fractures would therefore appear to be a sensible option in such cases. There is certainly some

Table 6.3 Indications for open reduction and fixation of condylar neck fractures.

Absolute indications:

- Displacement of condyle into middle cranial fossa
- Impossibility of restoring occlusion without ORIF
- Lateral extra-capsular displacement.
- Invasion by foreign body (e.g. missile)

Relative indications:

- Bilateral fracture with associated mid-face fracture (particularly where one condylar fracture is dislocated or angulated)
- Bilateral fracture with severe open bite deformity
- Unilateral fracture with dislocation, overlap or significant angulation of the condylar head
- When inter-maxillary fixation is contraindicated for medical reasons

evidence from post-operative MRI studies that open reduction leads to better anatomical restoration of both the condyle and the articular disc. Possible indications for open reduction of condylar neck fractures are shown in Table 6.3.

There is debate on how much emphasis should be placed on the radiographic findings as a factor in open reduction. Although guidelines are becoming available on relative indications such as the degree of overlap of the fragments and angulation of the condylar head, these are still not fully agreed. If surgery is contemplated, early intervention is technically much easier than when it is deferred for a few weeks.

ORIF of a condylar neck fracture has in the past been regarded as technically difficult although many authors have reported satisfactory results. Earlier methods, which sometimes required special instrumentation, employed a submandibular approach to expose the fracture, combined with a classical pre-auricular approach to the TMJ if needed. Although there are still advocates of this technique, particularly if long lag-type screws from the lower border are used, most surgeons currently adopt a retromandibular or transparotid approach that gives good access for plate fixation. The retromandibular approach involves a short vertical incision through skin and subcutaneous fat 0.5 cm below the attachment of the ear. Blunt dissection proceeds in the same orientation, which is parallel to the lower division of the facial nerve, to reach the posterior border of the mandible, with careful identification and protection of any nerve branches if they are visualized. The pterygomasseteric sling and periosteum is incized at the posterior border to allow wide subperiosteal dissection (Fig. 6.15). The transparotid approach is a variation of this technique whereby the dissection proceeds anteriorly on the surface of the parotid fascia, prior to blunt dissection between the anticipated zygomatic and buccal branches of the facial nerve.

The most difficult aspect of any open approach to condylar fractures is reduction of the proximal fragment, particularly if there is fracture dislocation of the condyle. Inferior displacement of the ramus is usually needed and specialist instruments have been devised to facilitate this and give good exposure. Retrieval and stabilization of an anterior or medially displaced condylar fragment will often require the help of bone forceps, a bone hook or a traction wire attached to a screw temporarily inserted into the bone. If standard

miniplates are used for fixation it is generally advised that two must be placed to avoid relapse due to the continuing displacing forces of the medial pterygoid muscle (Fig. 6.16). This is not always technically possible, particularly in higher condylar neck fractures, and as a result a number of slightly heavier specially shaped plates have been developed for this purpose.

Using these ORIF approaches consistently good functional and anatomical reconstruction is possible and there is increasing evidence that selective open reduction improves outcome particularly in bilateral and/or displaced condylar fractures.

Endoscopic assisted repair

Minimally invasive endoscopic repair of condylar fractures has been reported to offer less morbidity and operating time, as well as quicker patient recovery. But

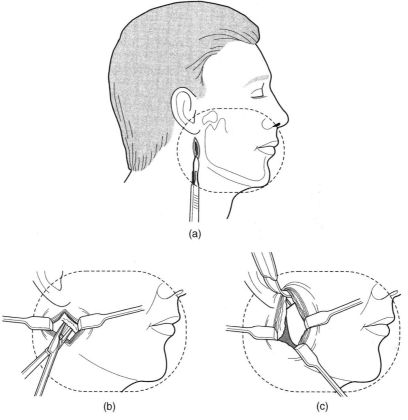

(a)

(b)　　　　　　　　　　　(c)

Figure 6.15 Diagram illustrating the steps in a retromandibular approach to the mandibular condyle. (a) 1.5–2.0 cm vertical incision just behind the posterior border of the mandible. (b) The cutaneous incision is essentially parallel to the main lower division of the facial nerve and subsequent blunt dissection to reach the mandible avoids damage to this structure. (c) Wide subperiosteal dissection exposes the fracture site. (See text for details.)

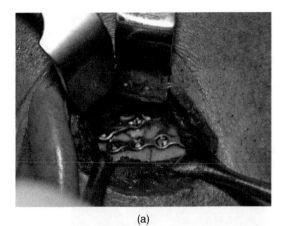

(a)

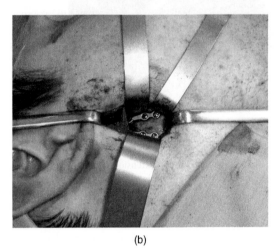

(b)

Figure 6.16 (a) Direct fixation of right condylar neck fracture using a retromandibular approach. The patient is supine with the earlobe to the left of the picture. Note two plates in position to resist displacing forces. (b) A similar technique using a slightly more anterior transparotid dissection. (Reproduced with kind permission of Springer Science+Business Media.)

like all developing techniques there is a learning curve. Case selection is very important, and the technique is reported to work best for low condylar fractures with lateral displacement of the upper fragment. Endoscopic repair is more difficult but not impossible for medially displaced fractures. Comminuted and high level fractures require considerable surgical skill and experience. The main advantages of the technique lie in reduced risks to the facial nerve and minimal scarring, compared with standard percutaneous approaches.

Major complications
Ankylosis of the temporomandibular joint
It has long been recognized that ankylosis of the temporomandibular joint can occur following trauma. Equally it is now clear that this is a very rare complication. The fact that ankylosis appears to be commoner in some parts of the world than in others has led to speculation that there may be a genetic predisposition among some racial groups. Fractures that involve the joint space, particularly in young patients, seem most prone to result in this complication although attempts to produce experimental ankylosis in primates have been notably unsuccessful.

Predisposing factors almost certainly include:
1 *Age*: the major incidence is below the age of 10 years.
2 *Type of injury*: intracapsular trauma with crushing of the condyle.
3 *Damage to the meniscus*: experimental work on large primates has shown that more restriction of movement occurs when an intracapsular fracture is accompanied by excision of the meniscus. Furthermore, remnants of the meniscus can be found in the medially displaced mass of bone, a finding that is common in human cases of bony ankylosis. Disruption of the meniscus is likely to occur in two particular types of fracture: a severe intracapsular compression injury or a fracture/dislocation (see Fig. 3.2 in Chapter 3 for an illustration of the mechanism of these types of injury).

Despite occasional suggestions in the literature there is no evidence that prolonged immobilization predisposes to either fibrous or bony ankylosis.

Disturbance of growth
A small proportion of children in which the fracture involves the condylar cartilage and the articular surface exhibit subsequent disturbance of growth. In some cases, fibrous or bony ankylosis of the temporomandibular joint is an additional complication. This reduces the normal functional movement of the jaw that further inhibits growth. In cases of post-traumatic arrested development of the condyle, coincident ankylosis is seen in a high proportion. There remains an ongoing debate as to whether or not the subcondylar region is a primary growth centre. In practical terms it does not matter whether this part of the mandible is a hormone-dependent primary centre for growth or an area where secondary bone formation takes place as

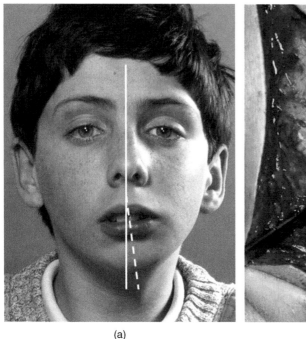
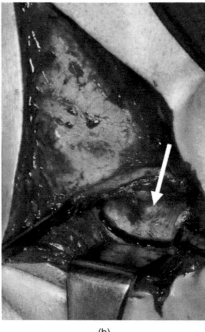

(a)   (b)

Figure 6.17 (a) Young patient who had sustained an intracapsular fracture of the left condyle some years previously. Note the smaller left hemi-mandible with deviation of the chin point to the left. This was associated with an increasing limitation in mouth opening. (b) Exposure of the left temporomandibular joint using a pre-auricular incision with a temporal extension. The condylar neck has been sectioned prior to removal of the deformed condylar head (arrowed). In this case the ankylosis was mainly fibrous.

the mandible develops within a functional matrix. The effect of damage is the same; failure of development of the condylar process and a smaller mandible on the affected side (Fig. 6.17).

Clinical management of condylar fractures: an overview

The methods of treatment of condylar fractures should be based on the clinical and experimental evidence outlined previously. Treatment should be designed to minimize subsequent functional disturbance of the articulation. The possible difficulties of open reduction and fixation need to be fully appreciated. Currently there are three treatment options:

1 Functional (conservative).
2 Indirect immobilization (IMF).
3 Osteosynthesis (ORIF).

Condylar fractures can be classified according to:
1 Age:
    Under 10 years.
    10–17 years.
    Adults.

2 Surgical anatomy:
    Involving joint surface: intracapsular.
    Not involving joint surface: extracapsular.
    High condylar neck.
    Low condylar neck.
3 Site:
    Unilateral.
    Bilateral.
4 Occlusion:
    Undisturbed.
    Malocclusion.

Children under 10 years of age

This group has been shown to be more likely to develop growth disturbance or limitation of movement than other groups. If malocclusion is present entirely as a result of condylar injury, it should be disregarded because spontaneous correction will take place as the dentition develops. Displaced condylar neck fractures will undergo full functional restitution in most cases.

Unilateral and bilateral fractures are treated in the same way. Treatment should be entirely functional where possible. Indirect immobilization by IMF may be indicated for control of pain but should be released after 7–10 days. Where an intracapsular fracture has been diagnosed careful follow-up and monitoring of growth is required and appropriate orthodontic treatment instituted if subsequent mandibular development is affected. Similarly, any sign of developing ankylosis will require surgical intervention.

Adolescents 10–17 years of age

The same principles apply to this group with some modification. If malocclusion is present the capacity for spontaneous correction is less than in the younger group. Malocclusion is therefore an indication for inter maxillary fixation for 2–3 weeks. The dentition at this stage is suitable for the application of bonded brackets and elastics, simple eyelet wires or arch bars. There is an argument for ORIF when there has been major displacement of the condyle as in a severe fracture dislocation.

Adults

Unilateral intracapsular fractures

The occlusion is usually undisturbed and the fracture should be treated conservatively without immobilization of the mandible. Occasionally slight malocclusion is noted, particularly when there is an associated effusion in the joint, in which case simple IMF can be applied for 2–3 weeks.

Unilateral condylar neck fractures

If the fracture is undisplaced or minimally displaced the occlusion will generally be undisturbed and no active treatment is necessary. A fracture/dislocation will often produce significant malocclusion due to shortening of the ramus height and premature contact of the molar teeth on that side. A low condylar neck fracture is probably best treated by open reduction in these circumstances. In the case of a high condylar neck fracture with extensive displacement and malocclusion a judgement needs to be taken on whether ORIF is technically possible. This will depend to some extent on the availability of special equipment and suitable plates, but more importantly on the skills and experience of the operator. If there is any doubt a safer option is to apply and maintain IMF for 3–4 weeks until stable bony union has occurred. In spite of restoring the occlusion by IMF relapse may take place when the fixation is removed and intermittent elastic IMF may be needed for a few weeks more. Any slight residual malocclusion can be corrected by a combination of occlusal adjustment and spontaneous adaptation. Extensive occlusal grinding or residual TMJ dysfunction is certainly not desirable and for this reason there is an increasing body of opinion in favour of ORIF.

Bilateral intracapsular fractures

The occlusion is usually slightly deranged in these cases. The degree of displacement of the two condyles may not be the same and it is best to immobilize the mandible for the 3–4 weeks required for stable union. It used to be thought that this would predispose to chronic limitation of movement but post IMF physiotherapy in the form of simple jaw exercises is effective in preventing this.

Bilateral condylar neck fractures

These fractures present the major problem in treatment. There is usually considerable displacement of one side or the other. Even if displacement is not evident when first seen, the fractures are inherently unstable and conservative functional treatment is usually contraindicated. Although the application of IMF will re-establish the occlusion, it will not reliably reduce the fracture on both sides. Operative reduction and fixation of at least one, and preferably both, of the fractures to restore the ramus height(s) is therefore desirable.

In the case of bilateral very high condylar neck fractures where operative reduction is likely to be difficult or occasionally technically impossible, IMF can be applied for up to 6 weeks. If robust arch bars are applied this will allow the use of intermittent intermaxillary elastics at night for several weeks after fixation is released. This technique may encourage functional remodelling.

Although ankylosis of the temporomandibular joint itself does not occur with condylar neck fractures, exuberant callus formation round grossly displaced fragments may cause extra-articular interference with joint excursion.

When bilateral fractures are associated with a major mid-facial fracture, operative reduction of both sides is desirable. It should be appreciated that this represents a considerable amount of operating time, even in skilled hands. Nevertheless modern materials and a retromandibular or transparotid approach make the procedure perfectly practicable. As mentioned previously, ORIF of a condylar neck fracture requires the fixation to be of adequate strength and a single standard miniplate is not sufficient, let alone anything smaller, because it will frequently fracture or dislodge within a few days. Two standard size mandibular miniplates should therefore always be inserted. Alternatively one of the custom designed condylar fracture plates can be used.

Fractures of the condylar region: synopsis

1 Fractures of the condylar region involve the temporomandibular joint either directly or indirectly.
2 Permanent disturbance of function of the TMJ is common when carefully looked for but is usually not significant. Fractures that involve the subcondylar area in children can occasionally lead to significant disturbance of growth. Fractures into the joint space can result in fibrous or bony ankylosis that appears to be more common in some racial groups than others.
3 All intracapsular fractures and all fractures in growing children should be treated conservatively. Immediate or early mobilization should be encouraged. However, if the occlusion is disturbed IMF is applied and maintained until stable union can be expected to be present.
4 Significantly displaced subcondylar fractures in adults, particularly when there are bilateral fractures, should be treated by ORIF.
5 Retromandibular or transparotid surgical approaches to the subcondylar region give rapid and sufficient access for the application of bone plates that must be of adequate strength.
6 Treatment of fractures of the condylar region in all age groups is still less than ideal and although guidelines exist they remain to be evaluated fully.

Fractures of the edentulous mandible

The physical characteristics of the mandible are altered considerably following the loss of the teeth. In effect, from the point of view of treatment, the edentulous mandible becomes a different bone. Following resorption of the alveolar process, the vertical depth of the denture-bearing area is reduced by approximately one-half and in some cases by considerably more. The resistance of the bone to trauma is further reduced by changes in the structure of the bone associated with the process of ageing. Together with age related changes in health and physiology, the denture-bearing area of the edentulous mandible is therefore not only more easily fractured, but also less well disposed to rapid and uneventful healing. In addition, the smaller cross-sectional area of bone at the fracture site and the absence of the stabilizing influence of teeth mean that the bone ends are more easily displaced and even after reduction the area of contact between them may be insufficient for healing to occur easily. The more atrophic the mandible the more significant these factors become.

It is not unusual to see bilateral fractures of the body of the edentulous mandible, each occurring near the posterior attachment of the mylohyoid diaphragm. Due to alveolar resorption the mylohyoid muscle in the edentulous jaw is attached relatively higher up on the lingual side than when the teeth are present. In addition, because there are no teeth to absorb some of the energy of impact, these fractures are often significantly displaced. These factors combine to create a situation whereby extreme downward and backward angulation of the anterior part of the mandible takes place under the influence of the digastric and the mylohyoid muscles. Extreme displacement may lead to respiratory distress, particularly in an elderly patient. This 'bucket handle' displacement peculiar to the thin edentulous mandible is illustrated in Fig. 2.3 (see p. 13).

However, the edentulous state does confer a few advantages. Fractures are, for instance, much less frequently compound into the mouth than when teeth are present. As a result if treatment is by closed reduction the risk of subsequent infection of the fracture is negligible. The absence of teeth means that precise anatomical reduction is not necessary as any inaccuracy is easily compensated by adjustment of dentures. For these reasons, many fractures in edentulous patients require no active treatment at all. If the fracture is simple with little or no displacement it will heal satisfactorily if the patient refrains from unnecessary active movements and adjusts to a temporary soft diet. Any subsequent discrepancy in the fit of the denture can be corrected in most cases by relining with or without occlusal adjustment.

In very elderly and infirm patients unfit for surgical intervention, the clinician should aim first and foremost for a stable pain free fracture site, achieved at minimal risk to the patient. Fibrous union alone may provide this result but occasionally this may, in turn, condemn the patient to a long or even permanent period when they are unable to wear dentures. A fibrous union in the body of the mandible will often calcify slowly over a period of up to 12 months. Distortion of the alveolus resulting from malunion is less of a problem than it used to be because patients may be able to have osseointegrated implants inserted to retain good functioning dentures.

With the ever increasing use of implant retained prostheses, a number of edentulous mandibular fractures may occur at the site of an implant fixture. Indeed, implants like unerupted teeth may predispose to fracture of the bone where they are located. In these circumstances an implant fixture would be treated in the same way as an unerupted tooth and will almost certainly have to be removed with the minimum of bone loss to facilitate healing.

Reduction

For the reasons already stated, precise anatomical reduction is not essential in fractures of the denture-bearing area. This is fortunate if closed reduction is used because it is frequently difficult when there is over-riding of the bone ends. Both closed and open reduction and subsequent fixation become more difficult as the mandible atrophies. The reduced cross-sectional area of the fractures of thin mandibles means that displacement occurs more readily and in this situation open reduction is the only reliable way to restore adequate bone contact. However, open reduction involves further disruption of the periosteal attachment, detrimental to repair of bone. Clinical judgement is required, the objective being to achieve sufficient bone contact and alignment, with the minimum direct operative interference at the fracture site.

Methods of immobilization

There is no doubt that the traditional treatment by means of closed reduction and Gunning-type splints has effectively been superseded by methods that employ open reduction and direct skeletal fixation. In older patients IMF is even less desirable than in younger age groups. Nutritional requirements become difficult to maintain and oral candidiasis commonly affects the oral mucosa causing considerable discomfort during the active treatment period. Possible methods of treatment are listed in Table 6.4.

Table 6.4 Methods of immobilization for fractures of the edentulous mandible.

---

a. Direct fixation (osteosynthesis):
    Bone plates
    Transosseous wiring
    Fixation supplemented by cortico-cancellous bone graft.
b. Indirect skeletal fixation:
    Pin fixation
    Custom external fixator
c. Inter-maxillary fixation (using Gunning-type splints):
    Used alone
    Combined with other methods

Direct fixation (osteosynthesis)
Bone plates

Bone plates are particularly useful for displaced fractures of the edentulous mandible. They allow the fracture to be stabilized without immobilization of the jaw as a whole. The patient is, as a result, more comfortable during the healing period. The mandibular plating systems described earlier in the chapter are in general applicable to edentulous fractures. Unlike the dentate mandible there is an increased risk of non-union in the edentulous state and it could be argued that compression plates might have a theoretical advantage. However, the reduced thickness and strength of bone in the edentulous mandible favours the use of non-compression miniplates rather than bulkier rigid or compression plates. Bone plates are easier to apply in the edentulous state than when teeth are present as there is no need to achieve the same degree of precision in the reduction of the fracture. Any discrepancy in the eventual occlusion of the pre-existing dentures is more easily corrected than when natural teeth are involved.

It is also easier and better to apply bone plates to the edentulous mandible than it is to insert transosseous wires, although both techniques carry an increased risk of damage to the inferior alveolar nerve in thinner mandibles. Wires require liberal exposure of the fracture site with extensive elevation of the periosteum, plus the fact that they do not achieve rigid fixation. With plates, exposure can be confined to one surface of the bone and the overall periosteal attachment is often considerably less disturbed. All plating systems require an adequate blood supply to achieve bony union and wide elevation of periosteum in the thinner mandible seriously compromises the blood supply to the fracture site.

Plates related to the denture-bearing part of the mandible are much more likely to require removal at a later date than those used in the ramus or in dentate fracture sites. Nevertheless some form of plating is currently the preferred method of fixation for the majority of edentulous mandibular body fractures. When first introduced resorbable plates appeared to have a potential advantage but at their present stage of development degradation takes place over a period of 2 years or more during which new dentures are likely to be needed. A metal plate removed electively is a better option.

Primary bone grafting

The ultra-thin mandible

Extreme atrophy of the edentulous mandible can occur to such an extent that the mandibular neurovascular bundle may come to lie above the bone covered only by soft tissue. While this is relatively uncommon and usually associated with old age, this is not always the case. Some female patients, particularly those suffering from premature osteoporosis and who have been edentulous from an early age, may have ultra-thin mandibles by the fifth decade. Fracture of the body of the mandible can result from minimal trauma and may even occur spontaneously. Treatment of such a fracture by ORIF may fail because the bone ends are difficult to reduce, further fragmentation may occur as the result of drilling and bone contact is minimal. These factors, together with the interference to the local periosteal blood supply, lead inevitably to non-union.

The panoral tomogram provides a rough but useful classification. If the depth of the thinnest part of the body of the mandible is less than 1 cm on the radiograph it should be classified as ultra-thin and therefore demand special treatment.

Primary bone grafting to stabilize and augment a fracture of the body of the ultra-thin edentulous mandible may be undertaken in selected cases. A 5 cm length of rib is obtained as an autogenous graft. The rib is split and the two pieces are placed one on each side of the fracture site, in the manner of a first-aid splint applied to a limb. The rib is then secured in place by means of self-tapping or lagged titanium screws that engage both buccal and lingual parts of the split graft. Alternatively, the rib halves may be lashed firmly together by several circumferential sutures or light wires, sandwiching the fractured bone ends between them (Fig. 6.18). Iliac bone

can be employed in a similar fashion but rib lends itself ideally to this technique.

Although this method of treatment may appear demanding for an elderly patient it is in practice often much less traumatic than supposed. Furthermore, the results achieved have been found to be consistently good and bony union is usually accomplished in even the most unfavourable of edentulous fractures. Postoperative morbidity at the donor site can be considerably reduced by controlled infusion of bupivacaine into the wound area through a fine catheter. After healing is complete the bulk of the mandible at the previous fracture site is increased, which in turn assists in the provision of a denture. This approach may be considered in treating any edentulous fracture of the body of the mandible where there is a significant risk of non-union.

Indirect skeletal fixation

Extra-oral fixation can be used in edentulous mandibular fractures in the same manner as for the dentate mandible. The method is occasionally of practical use in some pathological fractures due to bone neoplasms, or when there has been extensive comminution of a long segment, particularly if this involves the symphysis. However, since the advent of bone plates it has to be accepted that this method is mainly of historical interest.

IMF using Gunning-type splints

This is another method that has been effectively superseded by modern plating techniques but it will be mentioned here for completeness. Historically, the dental splint described originally by Gunning in 1866 was a vulcanite overlay of the natural teeth that he used as a splint for the fractured dentate mandible. A similar splint for the edentulous mandible consisted of a type of removable monobloc resembling two bite blocks joined together.

Gunning-type splints take the form of modified dentures with bite blocks in place of the molar teeth and a space in the incisor area to facilitate feeding. They are fixed to the jaws by circum-mandibular and maxillary peralveolar wires or screws, and IMF is then effected by connecting the two splints with wire loops or elastic bands (Fig. 6.19).

This far from ideal method, which is only ever indicated in simple fractures, is a technique that is all but obsolete. The splints become exceedingly foul during 4–6 weeks of fixation as a result of food stagnation

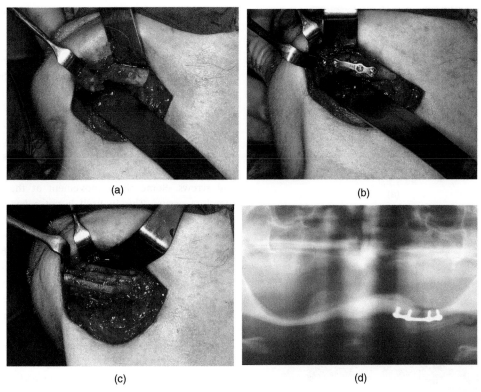

(a)   (b)

(c)   (d)

Figure 6.18 Primary bone grafting to fracture of a thin edentulous mandible. (a) Displaced fracture of left body exposed. (b) Reduction and alignment with the help of a small miniplate. This is insufficient for effective stable fixation because the screws only engage lightly in thin and atrophic bone. (c) Segments of split rib graft applied to superior and inferior surface and held in place with tightly tied circum-mandibular polydioxanone resorbable sutures. (d) Postoperative OPT showing reduction and stabilization with the help of the rib graft (faintly visible at the lower border). Healing was uneventful.

between the poorly fitting surface of the splint and the mucosa. This predisposes to *Candida*-induced stomatitis and infection of the retention wire tracks within the tissues. In the final analysis, Gunning-type splints are inefficient as a method of immobilization and provide poor control of mobile fractures, particularly when the mandible is very thin.

Fractures of the edentulous mandible: synopsis

1 In the edentulous mandible reduction and fixation is in the main required for fractures of the angle and body with a view to restoring an adequate denture-bearing area and avoiding facial deformity.

2 Because of the risk of non-union resulting from interference with the periosteal blood supply,

reduction should be accomplished with minimal exposure. Many undisplaced fractures require no active treatment.

3 Gunning-type splints have little, if any, modern application as a treatment modality.

4 The most effective form of osteosynthesis is by non-compression miniplates. In otherwise fit patients, open reduction and direct osteosynthesis is the method of choice. Inter-maxillary fixation should be avoided wherever possible.

5 When the mandibular body is less than 10 mm in depth, fracture treatment becomes difficult and non-union is more likely. It must be remembered that stable fibrous union may be an acceptable result in the very old or infirm patient.

6 The ultra-thin mandible may not unite satisfactorily with conventional methods of reduction and fixation

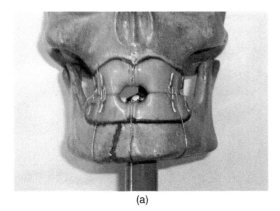

(a)

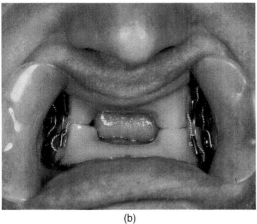

(b)

Figure 6.19 In the past many fractures of the edentulous mandible were treated by closed reduction and fixation with the help of Gunnings type splints. These are no longer in common use but are illustrated here for historical interest. (a) Model demonstrating how splints are held in place with circum-mandibular and per-osseous wires. (b) Clinical application.

and in these cases autogenous bone grafting as a primary procedure should be the method of choice where the patient's general condition permits.

7 Despite the previous comments, the best way to manage these sometimes difficult fractures is still not agreed and the literature can be confusing. A 2007 Cochrane Database review on this subject found that there was inadequate evidence to show better outcomes with any single approach over the other alternatives. Treatment is therefore based on the surgeon's experience and must be considered on a case-by-case basis. Close follow-up is advised.

Comminuted and complex mandibular fractures

In most maxillofacial units today, the overwhelming majority of low-energy mandibular fractures are managed using transoral miniplate osteosynthesis. Conceptually, this form of osteosynthesis using mono-cortical fixation is often referred to as 'load sharing'. This means that following repair, a proportion of the functional loading across the fracture is carried by the bones themselves and not entirely by the plates and screws. Some slight movement at the fracture therefore occurs. This in itself is not a bad thing; a small amount of loading across a fracture encourages 'micro-movement', which itself encourages healing. It is only when a fracture is overloaded that this becomes a problem. Any fracture that cannot be treated with load-sharing principles may be referred to as complex. This includes some pathological fractures, for example due to bone metastasis, and fractures resulting from high energy trauma.

Higher energy injuries to the mandible resulting in comminution are a difficult group of fractures to manage and are commonly associated with complications if inadequately repaired. Extensively comminuted fractures, such as occur following missile injuries, may involve a considerable area of mandibular bone. Perhaps surprisingly even where there are strong muscle attachments, such as over the ramus and angle, the amount of displacement of the comminuted segment may be remarkably little. This is explained by the fragmentation at the site of the muscle attachments. The small fragments are pulled away by the contracting muscle leaving the bulk of the comminuted bone relatively undisplaced. A significant proportion of the energy during impact is expended in associated soft tissue damage and many of these fractures are open (compound) and contaminated.

Multiple fragments, some often very small, are difficult to stabilize without using an excessive numbers of miniplates. The fragments are often difficult to manipulate and secure, while maintaining their soft tissue attachments and are therefore at risk of becoming loose or devitalized later on. All this results in a high risk of fragment necrosis, sequestration, non-union, infection and, in some cases, continuity defect. Successful management seeks to combine adequate immobilization and vascularization of the fragments while preventing subsequent infection.

Traditionally, management of these fractures used closed techniques, thereby avoiding periosteal stripping and further devitalizing the bone. However, these techniques do not guarantee adequate immobilization of all the fragments, although clinically they work well in selected cases. In recent years a more aggressive approach has been advocated with open reduction and rigid internal fixation. A number of studies have argued that maintaining the periosteal attachment is not as important as stabilizing the bony fragments and this is only possible if the fixation is rigid.

Two elements are essential for success:
1 The fixation needs to be fully load-bearing.
2 There must be absolute stability across the fracture.

Where this can be achieved small bone fragments can be replaced and fixed as free bone grafts leading to rapid bone healing and a lower rate of infection.

The choice of treatment therefore lies between maximizing the soft tissue attachments and vascularity by using IMF and/or external fixation or maximizing stability across the fragments by load-bearing osteosynthesis (see Fig. 6.3). Unfortunately, both are not possible in the same patient, although some surgeons make a compromise by using smaller miniplates, with less periosteal dissection, supplemented with lag screws and IMF.

With very high impact energies, such as blast injuries, it is often recommended to delay treatment for at least several days or longer. This enables non-vital tissue to be more easily identified when it can be excised as part of the definitive repair. Once the airway is secure and haemorrhage controlled, these injuries are no longer life-threatening and can wait while further imaging defines the extent of the fracture. Temporary IMF or external fixation can be used in the interim. (The management of high impact injuries is discussed further in Chapter 10.)

Factors affecting method of treatment of mandibular fractures: general summary

A number of interrelated factors determine the choice of a method of treatment. Some of these may be enumerated as follows:

1 The fracture pattern.
2 The skill of the operator.
3 The resources available.
4 The general medical condition of the patient.
5 The presence of other injuries.
6 The degree of local contamination and infection.
7 Associated soft-tissue injury or loss.

The simplest method of treatment is not necessarily synonymous with the best and maxillofacial surgeons need to be trained in all available skills to manage the patient under their care. Direct skeletal fixation without the need for total immobilization of the jaw has been shown to produce consistently good results. Such methods demand special skills and resources to match. Even with special skills the necessary surgical instrumentation may not be available, particularly in economically disadvantaged areas of the world. Most fractures of the mandible can still be successfully treated with a suitable selection of arch bars and 0.45 mm soft stainless steel wire and these traditional techniques should not be lightly discarded. It should be remembered that in fractures of the tooth-bearing portion of the mandible, the restoration of the occlusion is of prime concern and methods that rely at least in part on IMF consistently achieve this end.

Severely displaced or comminuted fractures of the mandible, many fractures of the condyle, and fractures of the ultra-thin edentulous mandible are all injuries of considerable complexity that tax the skills of even the most experienced maxillofacial surgeons. In any type of mandibular fracture more than one method of treatment may well be suitable and the eventual choice may depend on such factors as the general condition of the patient, the timing of the treatment of other injuries, the presence of infection and even the availability of access to an operating theatre.

Further reading

Al-Belasy FA. A short period of maxillo-mandibular fixation for treatment of fractures of the mandibular tooth-bearing area. *J Oral Maxillofac Surg.* 2005;63:953–956.

Champy M, Lodde JP. Mandibular synthesis. Placement of the synthesis as a function of mandibular stress [in French]. *Rev Stomatol Chir Maxillofac.* 1976;77:971–99.

Ellis E, Muniz O, Anand K. Treatment considerations for comminuted mandibular fractures. *J Oral Maxillofac Surg.* 2003;61:861–870.

Ellis E, Zide MF. *Surgical Approaches to the Facial Skeleton.* 2nd Revised Edn. Lippincott Williams and Wilkins, 2005.

Schneider M, Erasmus F, Gerlach KL, Kuhlisch E, Loukota RA, Rasse M, Schubert J, Terheyden H, Eckelt U. Open reduction and internal fixation versus closed treatment and maxillo-mandibulary fixation of fractures of the mandibular condylar process: a randomized, prospective multicenter study with special evaluation of fracture level. *J Oral Maxillofac Surg.* 2008;66:2537–2544.

Scolozzi P, Richter M. Treatment of severe mandibular fractures using AO reconstruction plates. *J Oral Maxillofac Surg.* 2003;61:458–461.

Van Sickels JE, Cunningham LL. Management of atrophic mandible fractures: are bone grafts necessary? *J Oral Maxillofac Surg.* 2010;68:1392–1395.

Wittwer G, Adeyemo WL, Turbani D, et al. Treatment of atrophic mandibular fractures based on the degree of atrophy – experience with different plating systems: a retrospective study. *J Oral Maxillofac Surg.* 2006;64:230–234.

CHAPTER 7

Treatment of fractures of the midface and upper face

The definitive treatment of fractures of the middle third of the facial skeleton will vary according to the pattern of injury. As with all fractures, treatment consists of reduction and alignment, with immobilization of the fragments until union has occurred. Not all midface fractures need active fixation following reduction however. For example, most simple nasal fractures and some zygomatic complex fractures will be stable after reduction without further surgical intervention.

Most fractures of the midface will obviously involve the paranasal sinuses. If possible, patients should be advised to avoid forceful nose blowing; not simply because of the likelihood of surgical emphysema, but also because of possible contamination of the orbit and facial soft tissues (Fig. 7.1). On rare occasions this can lead to orbital cellulitis, which is both a sight and life-threatening condition. Concern about the risk of infection, rare though it is, explains why prophylactic antibiotics are commonly prescribed following midface injury. Protagonists of this approach suggest that the presence of blood in the sinuses, compound injuries and soft tissue haematoma add to the risk. However, the evidence remains relatively weak and the routine use of antibiotic prophylaxis is a contentious issue in facial trauma.

In common with mandibular fractures, the preferred method of treatment for the majority of midface fractures involves open reduction and internal fixation (ORIF). Transosseous wiring can still be effective in certain situations but the versatility of the many semi-rigid plating systems available makes this technique the method of choice.

Since open reduction is often indicated the surgical approaches to the midface in common use will be described first before discussing treatment of the various types of fracture. Appropriate exposure can be achieved using a variety of incisions, all of which should have minimal cosmetic morbidity. Depending on the pattern of fracture, these incisions can be used singly or in combination. In practical terms exposure of the inferior, middle or superior aspects of the midface may be required. This in turn corresponds to access to the maxilla, the zygomatic complex and orbit or the fronto-nasal region (Table 7.1).

Surgical approaches to the midface and upper face

Occasionally, existing overlying facial lacerations may give suitable access, but carefully sited elective surgical incisions will usually provide the best exposure. Gross swelling is common within a few hours of injury and surgery is often better delayed until this settles. In the presence of gross oedema aesthetically acceptable approaches to the periorbital and nasoethmoidal regions in particular are very difficult owing to the turgor of the tissues and loss of the normal surgical planes.

Incisions for surgical exposure of the maxilla
Vestibular
An intraoral vestibular incision through the non-keratinized mucosa overlying the alveolar process, followed by sub-periosteal elevation, gives excellent access to most of the antero-lateral aspect of the maxilla. A relatively limited unilateral incision is all that is required to expose the base of the zygomatic buttress, whilst a molar to molar incision gives access to the whole maxilla from the Le Fort I level to the inferior

Fractures of the Facial Skeleton, Second Edition. Michael Perry, Andrew Brown and Peter Banks.
© 2015 John Wiley & Sons, Ltd. Published 2015 by John Wiley & Sons, Ltd.

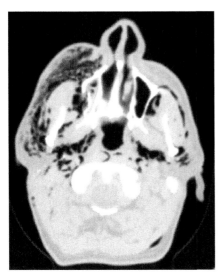

Figure 7.1 Axial CT scan showing extensive extravasated air in the soft tissues of the face (surgical emphysema) as a result of vigorous nose blowing following a fracture involving the paranasal sinuses.

Table 7.1 Surgical approaches to midface and upper face fractures.

1 Incisions for surgical exposure of the maxilla
  a. Vestibular
  b. Palatal
  c. Midface degloving procedure
2 Incisions for surgical exposure of the zygomatic complex and orbit
  a. Supero-lateral orbital rim
      Lateral eyebrow
      Supratarsal fold
      Extended preauricular
      Coronal and hemi-coronal (scalp flap)
  b. Lateral orbital rim, body and arch of zygoma
      Lateral canthal ('crow's foot crease')
      Extended preauricular
      Coronal and hemi-coronal (scalp flap)
  c. Inferior orbital rim and orbital floor
      Midtarsal or orbital rim
      Subciliary ('lower blepharoplasty')
      Transconjunctival (with or without lateral canthotomy)
  d. Medial orbital wall
      Paranasal (Lynch incision)
      Transcaruncular (+/- transconjunctival approach)
3 Incisions for surgical exposure the frontonasal region
  a. Local skin incisions (forehead, paranasal or nasal bridge)
  b. Coronal (bi-temporal scalp flap)

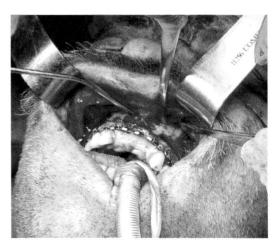

Figure 7.2 Intraoral vestibular incision used to expose the whole anterolateral aspect of the maxilla prior to bone plating. (Reproduced with kind permission of Springer Science+Business Media.)

orbital rims (Fig. 7.2). The subperiosteal dissection may be slightly more difficult than normal due to oedema and displacement of the bone segments. Comminution of the antral wall and base of the zygomatic buttress is common in zygomatic and Le Fort fractures and small bone fragments may be lost during the dissection as a result of periosteal detachment. This needs to be allowed for when placing miniplates.

Palatal

In severe facial injuries there may be a midline split of the maxilla. It is important to recognize this if the occlusion is to be restored correctly. If necessary a short miniplate can be placed across the fracture through a small sagittal palatal incision (Fig. 7.3), although with significantly displaced fractures the palatal mucosa is often lacerated. Ideally this incision should be to one side of the fracture to minimize the chance of an oro-nasal fistula developing. It is advisable to avoid raising a full mucogingival palatal flap since this, in combination with a vestibular incision, will seriously compromise the blood supply to the mobile maxillary segments.

Midface degloving procedure

This is rarely indicated in facial trauma but may have a limited use in the exposure of some Le Fort II type fractures. The technique combines an intraoral vestibular approach with degloving of the lower half of the nose

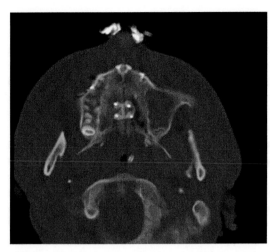

Figure 7.3 CT scan showing a midline split of the palate repaired with an H-shaped miniplate to restore normal maxillary width. Access to this area can be through a pre-existing palatal laceration or a judiciously placed incision. A full palatal flap should be avoided if a vestibular incision is also required. (Reproduced with kind permission of Springer Science+Business Media.)

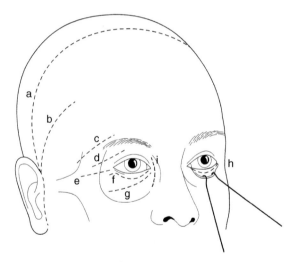

Figure 7.4 Diagram illustrating various incisions used for surgical access to the orbito-zygomatic region. (a) Coronal or hemi-coronal. (b) Extended preauricular. (c) Lateral brow. (d) Supratarsal fold. (e) Lateral canthus. (f) Subciliary. (g) Midtarsal. (h) Transconjunctival. (i) Paranasal.

to allow wide exposure of the whole maxilla including the nasal skeleton. Bilateral inter-cartilaginous incisions between the alar and lateral cartilages are made as for a rhinoplasty. The skin is elevated over the lateral cartilages and nasal bones and a transfixion incision

extended along the dorsal and caudal aspects of the septal cartilage to detach the columella. The intraoral vestibular incision is then used to expose the nasal spine and piriform aperture. The nasal mucosal attachment to these structures is divided to allow the premaxillary dissection to join the transfixion incision. Retraction of the soft tissues with further wide sub-periosteal dissection to the inferior orbital rim will allow complete exposure of the central midface skeleton. At the end of the procedure careful re-draping and suturing of the intranasal incisions is carried out and a nasal splint applied to minimize haematoma formation.

Incisions for surgical exposure of the zygomatic complex and orbit (Fig. 7.4)

Approaches to the supero-lateral orbital rim (fronto-zygomatic suture)

Lateral eyebrow

This straightforward approach to the fronto-zygomatic suture for the internal fixation of zygomatic fractures is less popular than it once was because of possible scarring. The exact placement of the incision is a matter of choice. It is usually sited just above the outer third of the eyebrow (Fig. 7.5), but can be placed within or just below it. Contrary to what may be supposed scars within the eyebrow are often the most obvious with the added risk of damaging the hair follicles. Sharp and blunt dissection to the supero-lateral orbital rim will expose the fracture site. Incision of the periosteum and subperiosteal dissection is normally started on the intact zygomatic process of the frontal bone and continued laterally. If there is separation or over-riding of the bone ends, probing and dissection with the points of a pair of sharp scissors will often facilitate location of the corresponding displaced frontal process of the zygoma.

Supratarsal fold

Although lateral brow incisions usually heal well they can leave a visible scar, which is most noticeable in young people. The supratarsal fold approach, sometimes inaccurately called the 'upper blepharoplasty' incision, gives an excellent cosmetic result and good exposure of the fronto-zygomatic suture. The skin incision is made just below the supero-lateral aspect of the orbital rim in the depth of the supratarsal recess (Fig. 7.6). The inherent mobility of the upper eyelid skin allows the tissues to be retracted laterally and subcutaneous

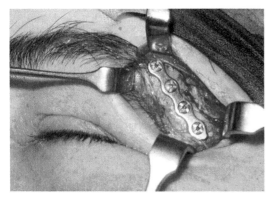

Figure 7.5 A straightforward approach to the frontozygomatic suture region is through an incision just above the lateral aspect of the eyebrow. Although commonly used it can leave a visible scar, particularly in young people.

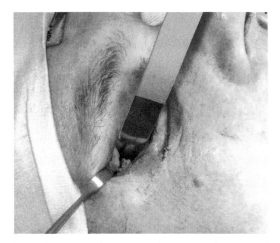

Figure 7.6 Supratarsal incision used to expose a fracture in the region of the right fronto-zygomatic suture. The laxity of the soft tissues of the upper eyelid region allows enough retraction to give wide exposure and the scar is essentially invisible. (Reproduced with kind permission of Springer Science+Business Media.)

dissection can then be carried out to the bone, which is exposed as in the lateral brow approach.

Approaches to the lateral orbital rim, body and arch of zygoma

Lateral canthal

The lower part of the lateral orbital rim or the body of the zygoma will usually be fractured in comminuted injuries. In this situation exposure of the fracture sites can sometimes be made through an incision in a suitable

skin crease lateral to the eye ('crow's foot' crease). It is much more usual, however, to combine this as an extension of a subciliary or transconjunctival incision as described below to give the wide exposure of the infero-lateral rim and body that is needed in this clinical situation.

Extended preauricular

Exposure of the whole zygomatic arch and the lateral aspect of the orbital rim can be obtained through this incision (Fig. 7.7). A short pre-auricular limb is combined with a curvilinear temporal incision extended well forward at an angle within the hairline. Dissection of the skin flap begins superficial to the deep temporal fascia. Approximately 2 cm above the zygomatic arch the fascia splits into two layers, one passing to the lateral aspect and one to the medial aspect of the arch. A variable amount of areolar tissue and fat is found between them. In order to avoid damage to the temporal branches of the facial nerve the dissection should proceed in the pocket between these two layers since the nerve lies lateral to the arch, and hence superficial to the lateral layer. Once the arch is reached, the periosteum is incised keeping to the medial side and then stripped forward to give the exposure required. Wider exposure of the body may necessitate a longer pre-auricular limb to allow the flap to be retracted well forward. Alternatively a full hemi-coronal flap should be considered (see below).

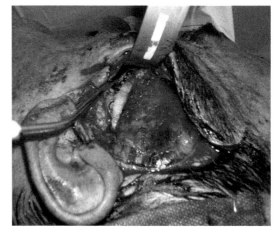

Figure 7.7 An extended preauricular incision showing the exposure achieved for repair of fractures involving the left zygomatic arch and inferior aspect of the lateral orbital rim. (Reproduced with kind permission of Springer Science+Business Media.)

Approaches to the inferior orbital rim and orbital floor

Surgical exposure of the orbital rim via an incision in the lower eyelid is by no means a standardized procedure and the terminology can be confusing. The skin incision can be at various levels and the subsequent dissection can be superficial or deep to the orbicularis muscle (Fig. 7.8).

To some extent the detail is a matter of preference but should take account of a number of factors:

1 Eyelid skin is very thin and needs to be handled with extreme care to avoid tearing and to minimize contusion of the skin flap. Extensive dissection superficial to the orbicularis muscle will increase this risk.

2 The incision should be designed to lie within the actual eyelid skin. Cosmetically unacceptable scarring will result if it is sited too low on the cheek skin.

3 An approach that is essentially deep to orbicularis appears to reduce the risk of transient or permanent ectropion.

4 A stepped approach through the skin, orbicularis and periosteum is reported to facilitate repair and prevent scar tethering.

5 Ideally, the incision through periosteum should be made on the anterior aspect of the orbital rim in order to avoid the insertion of the orbital septum along the orbital margin. Breaching this septum will lead to troublesome herniation of fat.

6 Oedema and periorbital haematoma will obscure the normal tissue planes and make dissection more difficult. If possible, it is advisable to delay surgical exploration until the swelling has settled.

Midtarsal

This is probably the easiest approach to the inferior orbital margin for the less experienced surgeon and the healed scar is rarely visible in the adult eyelid. The incision is placed in a natural crease approximately half way between the lash margin and the orbital rim (Fig 7.8a). It is important to design the incision in an oblique fashion starting closer to the lid margin medially and curving lower laterally. This facilitates lymphatic drainage and will prevent prolonged lymphoedema of the lower eyelid. Minimal skin dissection is carried out prior to division of the orbicularis at a slightly lower level. Dissection then proceeds superficial to the septum to reach the orbital rim.

Subciliary

The risk of post-operative oedema and the minor cosmetic problems of the midtarsal incision can be minimized by using a subciliary incision, sometimes called a lower blepharoplasty incision. This is placed in a suitable skin crease parallel to the free edge of the lid 2–3 mm away from the margin (Fig. 7.8b and c). The skin is dissected from the superior part of the orbicularis with care and the muscle is penetrated at a lower level. A short pre-septal dissection will expose the anterior aspect of the orbital rim and the periosteum is then incised and elevated. An advantage of this particular approach is that it can be combined with an extension in a lateral skin crease to achieve exposure of not only the floor but also the lateral wall of the orbit and even the body of the zygoma. It is technically more difficult than the midtarsal approach however and a possible disadvantage is the

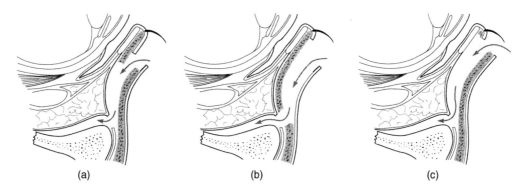

Figure 7.8 Diagram to illustrate various approaches to the inferior orbital rim using eyelid skin incisions. (a) Midtarsal incision with stepped post-orbicularis dissection. (b) Subciliary incision with pre-orbicularis dissection. (c) Subciliary incision with post-orbicularis dissection.

reported higher risk of ectropion. This probably relates to the more extensive pre-orbicularis skin elevation rather than the level of the incision on the eyelid itself. Most cases of post-operative ectropion settle with time and elective correction should not be considered for at least six months.

Transconjunctival

A conjunctival approach through the lower fornix has the obvious advantage of an invisible scar and avoids undermining of the lid skin. First described for cosmetic blepharoplasty it was later advocated for use in craniofacial surgery and orbital fractures. The dissection can either be post-septal, which is technically easier, or

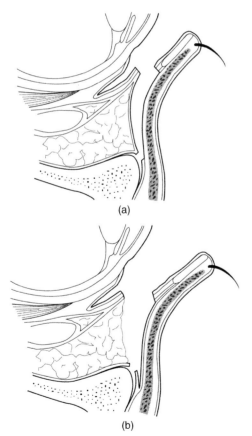

(a)

(b)

Figure 7.9   Transconjunctival approach to the inferior orbital rim. (a) Pre-septal dissection that minimizes herniation of orbital fat into the operative field. (b) Post-septal dissection that is considered technically easier.

pre-septal. The latter prevents unwanted herniation of fat into the surgical field (Fig. 7.9).

The transconjunctival incision is sometimes criticized for the limited access it provides beyond the inferior orbital rim but wide access can be achieved by the addition of a lateral canthotomy. This simple manoeuvre transforms the technique into a versatile single incision approach to the infraorbital rim, orbital floor, lateral wall and lateral rim, sometimes as far as the fronto-zygomatic suture. It is an excellent approach if the need for direct fixation at both the fronto-zygomatic suture and the inferior orbital margin is anticipated. The avoidance of skin and muscle incisions on the lower lid is a major benefit and ectropion or entropion are rarely seen.

If the canthotomy is performed first it will release the lower lid for easier access for the conjunctival part of the incision. One end of a pair of sharp iris or canthotomy scissors is placed in the recess of the lateral fornix and a clean cut of approximately 5 mm is made through the skin and mucosa (Fig. 7.10a).

The lid is then everted with traction sutures or skin hooks and, following the injection of a small amount of local anaesthetic with adrenaline, the conjunctiva and orbital septum are incised 2–3 mm inferior to the tarsal plate from just lateral to the lacrimal punctum to the lateral fornix. This manoeuvre is often more easily done by undermining from lateral to medial in the pre-septal plane prior to division of the conjunctiva (Fig. 7.10b). Once the conjunctival tissue has been incised it can be retracted with the help of elevation traction sutures (Fig. 7.10c). Dissection then proceeds deep to the orbicularis muscle to reach the orbital rim. The periosteum is incised and wide stripping of the periorbita from the floor and lateral wall can then be carried out to allow exposure of the infero-lateral aspect of the orbit (Fig. 7.10d).

At the end of the procedure the periosteum at the inferior rim is repaired if possible with a minimal number of sutures. Repair of the conjunctiva is not essential and may lead to increased post-operative chemosis. Care must be taken to restore the lateral canthal area, however. A fine slowly resorbing suture is used to repair the canthal tendon. Two fine sutures are then used to approximate the white and grey lines of the upper and lower lids at the lateral fornix. The edges of the canthotomy skin incision normally lie passively

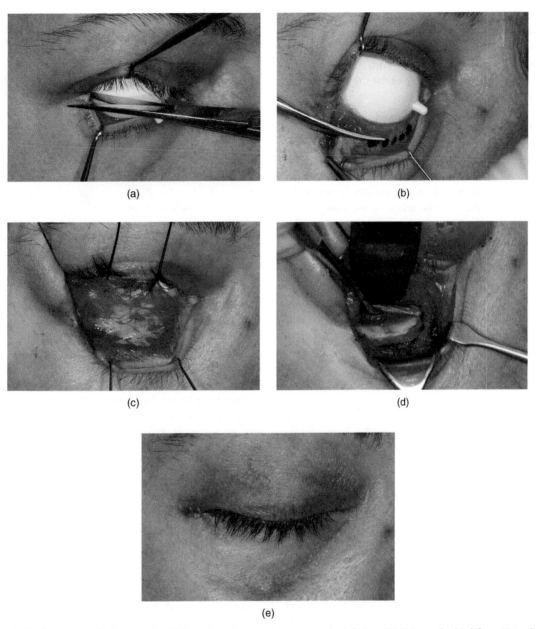

Figure 7.10 Transconjunctival approach with lateral canthotomy for access to the inferior orbital rim and orbital floor. Note globe protection by insertion of a soft eye shell. (a) Insertion of scissors into the lateral fornix prior to division of skin and lateral canthus. (b) Conjunctiva being divided by scissors after undermining in the pre-septal plane along the marked incision line. (c) Elevation of the conjunctival mucosa with the help of traction sutures. (d) Incision of periosteum over the orbital rim and initial stages of elevation of the periorbita to expose the orbital floor. (e) Closure of lateral canthotomy skin incision with two fine resorbable sutures. (Courtesy of Kenneth Sneddon, Queen Victoria Hospital, East Grinstead.)

together and simply require one or two sutures or an adhesive strip (Fig. 7.10e). Formal suspension of the canthus to the lateral rim is not needed unless a coronal approach has been combined with this procedure resulting in complete stripping of the orbito-zygomatic periosteum.

Approaches to the medial orbital wall
Paranasal

The classical and fairly straightforward approach to the medial orbit is through a small curved incision over the frontal process of the maxilla between the medial orbital rim and the bridge of the nose (Lynch incision. See Fig 7.8i). Subperiosteal dissection with infero-lateral displacement of the medial canthal structures and lacrimal sac allows access to the medial wall. Cautery and division of the anterior ethmoidal artery will facilitate wider exposure. The main problem with this approach is a visible scar with a high incidence of webbing due to secondary contracture. Z-plasty modifications have been described in an attempt to minimize this but a transcaruncular approach is now generally preferred.

Transcaruncular

Although it can be used on its own this approach is often designed as an extension of a lower fornix transconjunctival incision to give wide exposure of the medial aspect of the floor and the medial wall of the orbit. The upper and lower eyelids are retracted adjacent to the medial angle and the caruncle is gently grasped with fine forceps and pulled laterally. These steps flatten the area to improve visibility. The incision is made either just in front of, or across, the caruncle posterior to the lacrimal punctum. Blunt scissor dissection through the periorbital tissues just superficial to Horner's muscle (orbicularis) reaches the posterior lacrimal crest. A malleable retractor is inserted and the periorbita incized with a scalpel, or more easily by spreading the tips of sharp pointed scissors along the lacrimal crest. Careful sweeping dissection with a subperiosteal elevator exposes the medial orbital wall (Fig. 7.11). At the end of the procedure the periorbita is not usually closed. The conjunctiva and caruncular area are sutured using 6/0 resorbable sutures with buried knots.

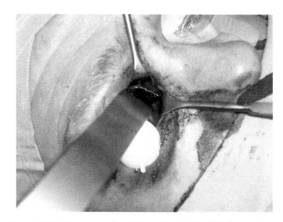

Figure 7.11 Exposure of medial wall of right orbit for titanium mesh repair by means of a transcaruncular approach. (Reproduced with kind permission of Springer Science+Business Media.)

Incisions for surgical exposure of the fronto-nasal region
Local skin incisions

A number of local incisions have been described for exposure of the nasal bridge and fronto-nasal region. These include an H-shaped incision across the bridge, Z-shaped incisions in the medial canthal areas, a midline vertical incision from the forehead across the glabella, and an extended W-shaped incision from above or beneath the medial aspect of one eyebrow across the nasal bridge to above or beneath the opposite eyebrow (see Fig. 7.27). Apart from any cosmetic shortcomings the problem with all these approaches is that the access is limited to a greater or lesser extent. Fracture lines may extend beyond the area of the surgical exposure and accurate reduction can be compromised as a result.

Coronal flap

The coronal, or bi-temporal, scalp flap gives unrivalled exposure of the whole of the upper part of the facial skeleton and has largely replaced the local incisions described earlier because of the superb visualization it gives of the frontal bone, naso-ethmoid region, superior orbital margins, lateral orbital margins and both zygomatic arches (Fig. 7.12). In common use by neurosurgeons for many years for craniotomy procedures, it was later adapted for craniofacial procedures and Le Fort III osteotomies, and soon became an established

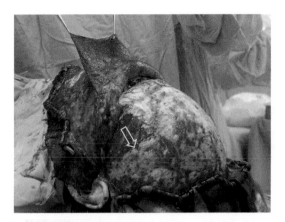

Figure 7.12 Coronal scalp flap raised to expose and plate orbito-naso-frontal fractures. A separate pericranial flap has been raised for protection of any anticipated anterior cranial base repair. Note also the oblique incision through the deep temporal fascia (arrow) to allow dissection superficial to the muscle to avoid damage to the frontal branch of the facial nerve. (Reproduced with kind permission of Springer Science+Business Media.)

method of treating craniofacial injuries and other complex facial trauma.

The incision is sited within the hairline. Laterally it extends into the preauricular region to allow complete exposure of the upper facial skeleton. In males, for cosmetic reasons, the incision should be sited over the vertex, to take account of possible later recession of the hairline. If no neurosurgical procedure is planned shaving of the head is unnecessary, but removal of a narrow strip of hair will facilitate the skin incision and closure.

Dissection is carried out in the virtually bloodless plane of subaponeurotic loose areolar tissue to a level just above the fracture area. Incision of the pericranium and subperiosteal dissection then exposes the upper third of the facial skeleton, although the supraorbital nerves have to be freed from their canals by careful peripheral osteotomy of both foramina with a small sharp osteotome before full exposure of the orbits and naso-ethmoid area is possible. Lateral elevation follows the technique described previously for an extended preauricular approach to the zygomatic arch.

A different approach should be used in frontal bone and orbital roof fractures, particularly if joint neurosurgical treatment is planned. In this situation a large pericranial flap should be raised from the outset in case it is needed to reinforce a dural repair or to cover any bone grafts of the anterior cranial base. At the end of the procedure drains are inserted and the scalp is closed in two layers.

Treatment of midface fractures

Fractures of the nasal bones

The vast majority of nasal fractures can be treated by closed manipulation and simple splinting. It is advisable to wait 5–10 days before reduction for the swelling to subside since this allows a clearer assessment of the injury.

More severe injuries, normally due to high energy frontal impact, often need open reduction. These grossly displaced fractures of the naso-orbito-ethmoid complex, which are frequently associated with other facial injuries, will be considered later.

Septal haematoma can sometimes develop as a result of bleeding into the subperichondrial space. This appears as a dark red swelling on the septum and results in partial nasal obstruction, usually within the first 24–72 hours. Untreated it can become infected leading to a septal abscess, with a risk of intracranial extension. Bilateral elevation of the perichondrium by blood or pus may also result in avascular necrosis with loss of cartilage and a septal perforation. Incision and drainage should be performed urgently under topical or local anaesthesia. The mucosa is incised over the area of greatest fluctuation, avoiding incision of the underlying cartilage. The clot is suction evacuated and the wound irrigated. Some authorities recommend excising a small piece of the mucoperichondrium and insertion of a drain to prevent premature closure of the incision and further accumulation of blood. The nose is then lightly packed. Broad-spectrum antibiotics should be administered and a specimen sent for culture.

Reduction

Simple nasal complex fractures with minimal displacement can be reduced under local anaesthesia. General anaesthesia with an oral endotracheal tube is still preferred by most surgeons and is definitely indicated when there is significant deformity, septal fracture or a risk of further haemorrhage. Manipulation of the nasal bones is a common yet often underappreciated procedure, which if performed poorly can result in residual deformity. The 'quick tweak' in the emergency or anaesthetic room is not surprisingly accompanied by poor outcomes, and more careful assessment is important. Failure to straighten the septum will inevitably result in some relapse, even if the nose appears straight at the end of the procedure. This results in part from the inherent elasticity of cartilage but also from overlap of the edge of a fairly common 'C-shaped' septal tear.

Some simple fractures can be reduced digitally. Otherwise, Walsham's and Asche's forceps are used for manipulating the fragments. One blade of the Walsham's forceps is passed up the nostril and the fractured nasal bone and associated fragment of the frontal process of the maxilla are secured between it and the external blade, which should ideally be padded with rubber or plastic tubing (Fig. 7.13). The fragments on each side are manipulated into their correct position. The vomer and the perpendicular plate of the ethmoid are then 'ironed out' with the Asche's septal forceps, using one blade each side of the septum after which, where possible, the septal cartilage is grasped and brought forwards and repositioned in its groove in the vomer. When the septum has been realigned the finger and thumb of one hand are used to compress the lacrimal bones and medial rims of the orbits to achieve a narrow bridge to the nose. Finally, a fine sucker should be passed down each of the nares to ensure that they are clear and that the patient has a patent nasal airway.

If the nasal bones are severely comminuted it may be possible to mould the nose into shape between the thumb and forefinger, or by applying a thumb along each side of the nose and squeezing. Such fractures tend to be much less stable after reduction and may well be part of a more extensive naso-orbito-ethmoid injury that would be much better treated by open reduction.

Fixation

When the fracture is minimally displaced, it may be unnecessary to splint the nose following reduction. Usually, however, some sort of splint fixation is advisable.

There are a number of custom made malleable or thermoplastic supports available although some surgeons still use a plaster-of-Paris splint. This consists of 6–8 layers of plaster-of-Paris bandage cut to produce a

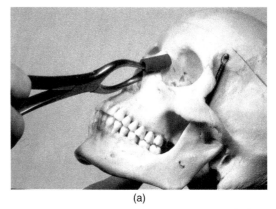

(a)

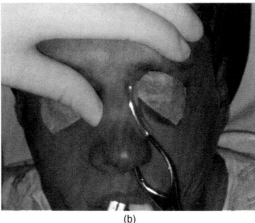

(b)

Figure 7.13 (a) Skull model and (b) Clinical case to show the position of Walsham's forceps when reducing a nasal fracture. The external blade is usually padded for added skin protection. (Reproduced with kind permission of Springer Science+Business Media.)

strip of plaster across the bridge covering either side of the nose, with an extension up to the forehead.

The preferred splint is moulded into place taking care to include the important medial canthal area. When it is firm it is fixed into position with strips of adhesive tape across the forehead and across the nasal bridge. A light nasal pack can be placed for 24 hours to help haemostasis but care must be taken to avoid over-packing and displacement of the nasal bones.

Ideally a fresh, accurately fitting splint should be applied a few days later when the post-operative oedema over the nasal region has subsided. A nasal splint should be left *in situ* for about 10–14 days in total. The aim of a splint is to help protect and maintain an already adequately reduced and stabilized fracture.

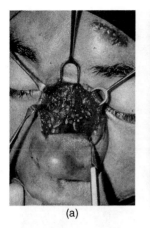 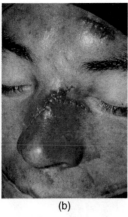
(a)   (b)

Figure 7.14 (a) Internal fixation of a comminuted nasal bone fracture made possible by an overlying laceration. (b) Restoration of nasal form and soft tissue repair.

ORIF of isolated nasal fractures is a procedure that is rarely advocated, probably because closed reduction is usually satisfactory. Nevertheless there are indications in selected cases particularly if there is an extensive overlying laceration (Fig. 7.14). Open reduction is more often indicated when the nasal bone fracture is part of a more complicated naso-orbito-ethmoid injury as will be discussed later below.

Fractures of the zygomatic complex

Zygomatic complex fractures with minimal displacement that are not causing symptoms do not necessarily require treatment. The indications for treatment are as follows:

1 To restore the normal contour of the face both for cosmetic reasons and to re-establish skeletal protection for the globe of the eye.
2 To correct diplopia.
3 To remove any interference with the range of movement of the mandible.
4 When pressure on the infraorbital nerve results in significant numbness or dysaesthesia.

Cosmetic deformity alone is more significant in some patients than others. Occasionally an obviously displaced zygoma is left untreated if the patient is elderly and a poor operative risk. At the other end of the scale even a minimally displaced fracture should ideally be elevated in a young, fit patient to restore contour and minimize the problems of late collapse.

Reduction

Surgical reduction of the displaced zygomatic complex becomes increasingly difficult with the passage of time. If necessary the operation can be delayed for up to 10 days to allow the swelling to settle. After two weeks the displaced bones start to become bound down by organizing scar tissue but it is still better to attempt primary correction rather than to settle for secondary reconstruction. In practice reduction can usually be achieved, although with some difficulty, up to 6 weeks after injury and occasionally even longer.

Many zygomatic complex fractures are stable after reduction without any form of fixation, particularly where the displacement is essentially a medial or lateral rotation round the vertical axis without separation of the fronto-zygomatic suture. Recent fractures tend to be more stable than those that are more than 2 weeks old. Fractures in which there is disruption of the frontozygomatic suture and those that are extensively comminuted are usually unstable after reduction.

Indirect reduction of a zygomatic fracture can be carried out by a temporal, percutaneous or intraoral approach.

Temporal approach

The temporal approach (Gillies approach) is popular and straightforward. The operation depends on the fact that the deep temporal fascia is attached along the superior surface of the zygomatic arch, whilst the temporalis muscle passes beneath the arch to be attached to the coronoid process and anterior ramus. Therefore, if an incision is made in the hairline in the temporal region and the temporal fascia is incised, it is then easy to pass an instrument superficial to the surface of the temporalis muscle and deep to the zygoma. The zygomatic bone or arch can then be elevated into a correct position (Fig. 7.15).

An oblique 2 cm incision is made within the hairline between the bifurcation of the superficial temporal vessels. The temporalis fascia is exposed and incised and a Rowe's or Bristow's elevator passed down beneath the zygomatic bone that is then elevated back into position. The position of the bone is confirmed by palpation of the infraorbital rim and the cheek prominence using the uninjured side for comparison. When palpating the reduced position it is important to relate the prominence of each zygomatic body to a common point distant from the bone, such as the glabella region, since periorbital

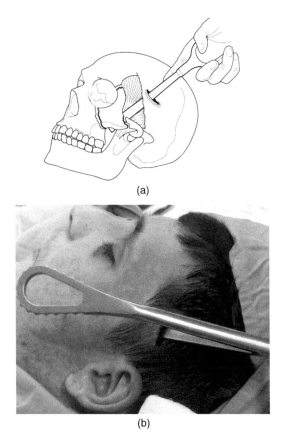

(a)

(b)

Figure 7.15 Gillies temporal approach for reduction of a fractured zygoma. (a) Diagram to illustrate how a zygomatic elevator (Bristow's) is inserted through an incision in the temporal fascia and passed superficial to the temporalis muscle to lie beneath the deep surface of the zygoma. (b) Clinical case using the same technique performed with a Rowe's elevator. (Reproduced with kind permission of Springer Science+Business Media.)

soft tissue swelling on the fractured side can give a false impression. When a satisfactory stable reduction has been obtained the temporal fascia and skin are sutured.

The Gillies approach is one the most versatile methods of indirect reduction. It is simple to perform and gives excellent control of the fractured zygomatic complex during all stages of reduction.

Percutaneous approach

This rapid method is most useful in non-comminuted fractures with medial displacement and no distraction of the fronto-zygomatic suture. A number of hook ended instruments have been designed for this purpose. The location of the stab incision for insertion of the hook

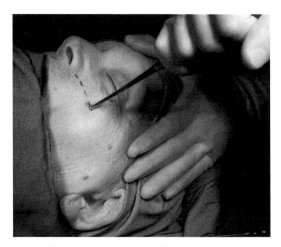

Figure 7.16 Depressed fracture of the left zygoma being elevated with the aid of a malar hook. The point of skin penetration is at the intersection of a horizontal line extending from the alar rim and a vertical line dropped from the lateral canthus. (Reproduced with kind permission of Springer Science+Business Media.)

elevator is found at the intersection of a perpendicular line dropped from the outer canthus of the eye and a horizontal line extending posteriorly from the alar rim of the nostril (Fig. 7.16). The point of the instrument is kept in close contact with the under-surface of the body of the zygoma and traction is applied to reduce the fracture. A single fine suture is all that is required to close the wound that is virtually invisible when healed.

Intraoral

Although this technique has a long history, it is not actually widely practised. An incision is made in the upper buccal sulcus immediately behind the zygomatic buttress and a curved elevator is passed supra-periosteally to engage the deep surface of the zygomatic bone. Forward and outward pressure is exerted to reduce the fracture.

Fixation
Direct fixation

The use of the surgical approaches described earlier, together with the benefits of direct osteosynthesis, has resulted in a move towards ORIF of most midfacial fractures. ORIF has a number of advantages. Firstly, exposure of the fractures allows for accurate repositioning of the anatomy. Secondly, fixation with miniplates affords greater stability and confidence in the repair.

Although closed techniques still have an important role to play in management of fractures of the zygomatic the move towards ORIF has become increasingly popular. The aim is to fix at least one, and preferably two, of the fracture sites with the object of resisting the effect of masseteric and other displacing forces that may act on the unsupported reduction following closed elevation.

Exposure of the infraorbital rim should be avoided if possible in the treatment of most isolated zygomatic fractures because of possible unwanted complications, including the risk of injury to the infraorbital nerve. Fixation at this site is also the weakest of all the fracture sites. Nevertheless, the orbital floor is always involved in fractures of the body of the zygoma and, if there is evidence of soft tissue herniation into the antrum or significant displacement of the orbital rim infraorbital exposure may be necessary to access the orbit and/or repair multiple rim fragments. For very small thin fragments smaller microplates are available, as are mesh and special grid design plates for use in orbital floor repair.

The decision about which sites to explore and plate depends to some extent on the type of displacement. If there is no strong indication to explore the orbital floor a zygomatic buttress plate placed intraorally is the best first option, with or without a plate at the frontozygomatic suture (See Fig. 7.5). A buttress plate allows inspection of the accuracy of reduction in this critical area at the base of the zygomatic buttress (Fig. 7.17). It is possible to obtain what appears to be good reduction at the lateral and inferior orbital margins and still to have a poor result because of rotation around the vertical axis or medial displacement at the base of the zygomatic buttress. This in turn will mean that the postero-lateral orbital wall is poorly reduced with a failure to restore orbital shape and volume. Some unexpected late enophthalmos may be due in part to this mechanism.

If open reduction is planned from the outset it is usually possible to reduce the fracture through the incision used to expose the fronto zygomatic suture. If this proves difficult a Gillies temporal approach should be used as well to get maximum control. It sometimes helps to place a temporary wire at the reduced fronto-zygomatic suture that will still allow some movement as the other sites are explored and reduced. As with all fractures, zygomatic complex fractures need to be considered in three dimensions and a mistake at the first fixation site will be compounded at the others.

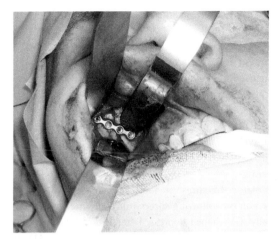

Figure 7.17 Fixation of fractured zygoma with the aid of a buttress plate. This is a critical site to check the accuracy of reduction in order that any residual rotation or medial displacement are avoided. (Reproduced with kind permission of Springer Science+Business Media.)

More recently resorbable plates and screws have been employed in the maxillofacial region, particularly in paediatric craniofacial surgery. Some of the earliest papers described the use of such plates in the fixation of zygomatic fractures. Although resorbable plates and screws appear to offer equivalent results in an animal model when compared to titanium plates, doubt remains about their real usefulness in adult clinical practice. They are technically more difficult to shape and require tapping of the screw holes; and their bulk precludes use at the infraorbital margin. The theoretical advantages of resorbable plates may seem obvious but any true benefits of these materials compared with titanium have yet to be proven and they are not in common use in facial trauma.

Indirect fixation

Indirect methods of fixation may have limited usefulness for rapid stabilization of an excessively mobile zygoma, or in reinforcing direct interosseous wire fixation, but the development of plating techniques has made them virtually redundant. They are mentioned here for completeness only.

One method that has been used in the past as a means of rapid stabilization is trans-antral internal pin fixation with a Kirschner wire. Similarly, a transnasal approach can be used in which the pin is inserted through the frontal process of the contralateral maxilla across the nasal cavity to engage the antral surface of the fractured zygoma.

Fractures of the zygomatic arch

Fractures of the zygomatic arch associated with fractures of the zygomatic complex usually reduce when the main zygomatic bone fragment is elevated into its correct position. ORIF is only required if there is gross comminution with displacement, significant overlap of the bone ends, or as part of the repair of complex multiple midface fractures.

Isolated fractures of the zygomatic arch are not uncommon following direct injury to the area. Classically a V-shaped depressed fracture occurs and may interfere with mouth opening (see Fig. 3.21, p. 41). In this situation the fragments should be reduced using a Gillies approach. A lighter instrument such as a periosteal elevator is usually sufficient to reduce the fracture, which clicks back in place easily if treated early enough. Fixation is normally unnecessary as the temporalis fascia attached along the superior aspect of the arch will provide the necessary immobilization. Fragments of the zygomatic arch will only be displaced downwards if their attachment to the temporalis fascia is stripped away. For this reason care should be taken to ensure that the elevator is passed deep to the arch on insertion. In the very rare event that temporary support of very mobile fragments is needed a balloon catheter can be passed beneath the arch through the Gillies incision and inflated with normal saline. Alternatively an external splint, such as a wooden tongue depressor or foam backed aluminium finger splint, can be placed over the arch and held in place with circumferential wires or heavy suture material. Open reduction and fixation is almost certainly a better option.

Fractures of the orbit

One or more walls of the orbit will always be involved in zygomatic complex, nasoethmoidal and high level maxillary fractures (Le Fort II and III type). In addition frontal bone and craniofacial fractures will frequently involve the supraorbital rim and orbital roof. Generally speaking the reduction of the main outer fracture fragments will restore the orbital anatomy, particularly in non-comminuted fractures, but it is important to identify those injuries that have resulted in significant disruption of the walls. In this situation, failure to restore the volume and shape of the orbit will result in post-operative enophthalmos and possible problems with ocular motility.

Although the floor is the most common part of the orbit to be involved in this way the advent of CT imaging has revealed that the medial wall is frequently involved as well, either in combination with the floor or as in isolated injury. This is to be expected when the fragile nature of the lamina papyracea is considered. Unsatisfactory results of treatment in the past may have been due in part to failure to recognize and correct medial wall or orbital roof defects, particularly if they are extensive. The management of fractures of the medial wall and roof will be considered later in the sections on naso-orbito-ethmoidal and craniofacial injuries but the more frequent clinical problem of orbital floor fractures demands special consideration.

Fractures of the orbital floor

It is important to recognize that two distinct types of orbital floor fractures can be identified:

1 Those occurring as part of the natural fracture pattern in fractures of the zygomatic complex or Le Fort II and III type fractures of the middle third of the face.
2 Those occurring as an isolated orbital floor fracture, either as a so-called 'blow-out' or rarely as a localized elevation or 'blow-in' fracture.

Enophthalmos resulting from herniation of orbital contents into the maxillary antrum can occur with either category, but diplopia due to interference with the action of the inferior rectus and inferior oblique muscles is more likely to be present in association with isolated orbital floor fractures.

Fractures in category 1 above are sometimes described in the literature as 'impure blow-out' fractures in contrast to the 'pure' blow-out fractures of category 2. These inelegant and inaccurate terms should be abandoned because the use of the description 'blow-out' presupposes a mechanism of injury. This is assumed to follow posterior displacement of the globe by blunt trauma or possibly deformation of the infraorbital rim with rupture of the floor. Conversely, it is obvious that the cause of most orbital floor injuries in category 1 is simply that they are part of the usual fragmentation of the facial bones that occurs in midface trauma.

Table 7.2 Possible complications of orbital floor exploration.

1 Intraorbital haemorrhage
2 Lower eyelid retraction and ectropion
3 Persistent oedema of lower eyelid
4 Persistent enophthalmos
5 Persistent globe depression
6 Persistent diplopia in vertical gaze
7 Tissue reaction to implant
8 Extrusion of implant
9 Infection and chronic fistula formation
10 Dacryocystitis
11 Blindness

Table 7.3 Indications and relative contraindications for orbital floor repair.

Indications

1 Significant restriction of eye movement (diplopia) with CT confirmation of entrapment
2 Significant enophthalmos
3 Large 'blowout' defect
4 Significant orbital dystopia

Relative contraindications

1 Visual impairment
2 Anticoagulant medication
3 Patient unconcerned
4 Proptosis
5 An already 'at risk' globe

To avoid confusion it is preferable to use the term 'isolated orbital floor fracture' for fractures in category 2 since this makes no assumption about aetiology but still defines a well-recognized clinical entity.

Treatment

The different opinions concerning treatment of orbital floor fractures expressed in the literature make objective evaluation extremely difficult. Although surgical exploration and repair is often carried out it is important to define the possible indications. The procedure should not be undertaken lightly as it is not without complication. (Table 7.2)

The indications for orbital floor exploration remain a controversial area of practice. While some fractures clearly require repair and others clearly do not, there remains a 'grey area' in which the need for surgery is largely a matter of opinion. This is partly due to the problem in defining what is considered to be clinically significant enophthalmos, and partly in accurately predicting when it will occur in any particular patient. In some patients there may be an obvious orbital floor defect, yet the amount of enophthalmos they eventually develop is less than anticipated. Furthermore, in many cases the patients themselves are not even aware of this. Therefore, the need for surgery has to be balanced against the small risks of potentially major complications.

When orbital fractures do require treatment and coexist with other fractures of the midface the latter must be repaired first. This is because safe orbital dissection and repair of orbital defects are dependent on repositioned key landmarks and a correctly positioned infraorbital rim to support an implant. This will not

be possible if the peripheral bones are significantly displaced.

In the absence of any significant diplopia surgical repair becomes largely a cosmetic procedure to prevent or treat enophthalmos. In this situation it should be remembered that there is a small risk that exploration could result in serious complications such as persistent post-operative diplopia or injury to the visual pathway. Although these risks are very small they need to be clearly discussed with the patient before surgery is agreed. The final decision in such cases is therefore largely a matter of clinician or patient preference, taking into account the risks and benefits of operating or not. Indications and relative contraindications for surgery are shown in Table 7.3.

If an orbital floor defect is large enough it will inevitably result in enophthalmos once swelling has fully settled. However, the precise dimensions of a 'large' blowout fracture as measured on CT imaging is unclear from the literature. A number of studies have looked into the relationship between orbital volume expansion and enophthalmos, but the findings are not consistent. It has been suggested that any defect greater than 1 cm × 1 cm will result in 'significant' enophthalmos. However, the site of the defect will probably have just as much bearing as the actual size, if not more. Defects involving the posteromedial bulge are more likely to have greater effect on globe position than similar sized defects sited more anteriorly.

Similarly opinions vary over what constitutes 'significant' diplopia. Diplopia is a relatively common early clinical finding after orbital trauma, often simply as a result of oedema affecting the extra-ocular muscles. Even if it is persistent in many patients it occurs only at the extremes of gaze. Diplopia is usually more of a clinical problem when looking downwards, for example when reading, but in some situations, such as drivers who need to check the rear view mirror or professional snooker and pool players, diplopia on looking upwards can be just as debilitating. Fortunately many cases of diplopia will resolve if managed non-surgically and eye movements are encouraged.

Deciding if and when to operate is therefore not always simple. In most cases a period of close follow up is necessary to determine if any of the initial symptoms and signs of diplopia are resolving or enophthalmos is getting worse. As mentioned earlier, since surgical repair always carries the small but devastating risk of blindness, or actually causing diplopia, a clear indication for surgery should always be established.

There is no doubt that the increasing use of CT scans to assess midface and orbital injuries gives a clearer picture of the damage caused to the orbital floor in an orbital injury. Orbital volumes can be measured using appropriate software after CT scanning and this can provide a valuable tool in the prediction of enophthalmos. CT also allows visualization of the other orbital walls, particularly the medial wall. Alteration in the shape of the floor, particularly loss of the normal upwardly convex contour of the posterior aspect, can result in an increase in volume that may be just as important as herniation of orbital fat as a cause of enophthalmos (Fig. 7.18). Nevertheless, it is always important to remember the adage 'treat the patient, not the X-ray'.

Where there is any uncertainty, a decision to operate will in most cases not need to be made before 7–10 days have elapsed. This allows time for oedema to subside and the true ophthalmic situation to be revealed. Ideally, all orbital floor fractures should be assessed both pre- and postoperatively in conjunction with an ophthalmic surgeon experienced in facial trauma. If there are clear indications for treatment primary intervention is essential since it is well recognized that delayed secondary treatment of fractures with diplopia and enophthalmos gives considerably inferior results. Common problems that may need addressing and the aims of surgical intervention are summarized in Table 7.4.

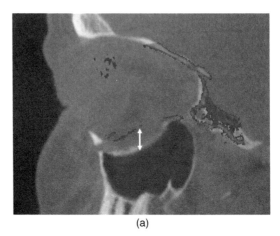

(a)

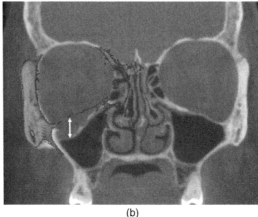

(b)

Figure 7.18 Sagittal (a) and coronal (b) CT scans of an isolated orbital floor fracture with 'mirror image' superimposition of the normal side (purple). The alteration in the shape of the orbital floor and the extent of the increase in volume is obvious as shown by the arrows. (Courtesy of Jeremy Collyer, Queen Victoria Hospital, East Grinstead.)

If there is disruption of the orbital floor with significant herniation on the CT scan, or functional problems due to soft tissue trapping, the orbital floor should be explored directly when the initial swelling has settled. A suitable lower eyelid or transconjunctival approach is made (see earlier) and the orbital contents are supported with a blunt malleable retractor while the orbital tissues are teased upwards through the defect in the orbital floor. A forced duction test will confirm that passive eye motility is restored completely.

There is one exception to delayed intervention. In children and young people with diplopia it is generally agreed that exploration should be performed as soon

Table 7.4 Aims of surgical intervention in orbital floor fractures.

Problem	*Aim of treatment*
Diplopia that does not resolve significantly during the first 10 days following injury	Restoration of ocular motility
Significant herniation of soft tissue into the antrum	Repair of orbital floor and correction/prevention of enophthalmos.
Incarceration of tissue sufficient to cause globe retraction and an increase in intra-ocular pressure on upward gaze	Restoration of function and prevention of fibrosis
Enophthalmos greater than 3 mm (i.e. evidence of significant increase in orbital volume)	Restoration of orbital volume and shape. Correction of enophthalmos.

as possible to prevent persistent problems. In this age group, due to the less brittle nature of the bone, the soft tissues are usually found to be trapped in a linear crack fracture rather than herniated into the antrum. If this is found to be the case it can sometimes be quite difficult to free the incarcerated tissue and sharp dissection across the floor of the orbit may even be required. Since no significant bone defect occurs in this type of fracture it is debatable whether repair of the floor is necessary.

In adults, gentle retrieval of the herniated soft tissues will more commonly reveal a defect in the medial aspect of the floor. It is important to delineate the margins of this defect, including the posterior edge, in order that any graft inserted will be well supported. It is always possible to identify the shelf of intact bone in the posterior aspect of the orbit even when there is gross disruption. The orbit is surprisingly deep and less experienced surgeons may be reluctant to explore beyond the equator of the globe. Anatomical studies suggest that the mean distance from the anterior lacrimal crest to the optic canal is 42 mm and it is considered safe to dissect for at least 25 mm posteriorly from the lateral aspect of the orbital rim and 30 mm from the anterior lacrimal crest (Fig. 7.19).

In larger defects better visualization can sometimes be achieved by performing a temporary osteotomy of the orbital rim (Fig. 7.20). This useful procedure considerably improves retrieval of herniated tissue and access to the posterior aspect of the orbital floor, and will facilitate safe dissection by enabling the posterior wall of the maxillary antrum to be followed superiorly until the residual bone ledge is found. When the bony defect has been defined it is covered with suitable implant or

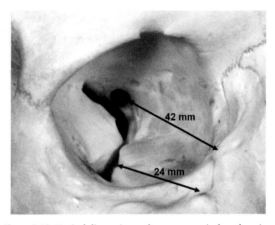

Figure 7.19 Typical dimensions relevant to surgical exploration of the adult orbital floor. Mean distance from anterior lacrimal crest to the optic foramen = 42 mm. Distance from infraorbital foramen to inferior orbital fissure = 24 mm. The depth of the orbit is often unappreciated by less experienced surgeons who may not explore far enough posteriorly to identify the intact bony ledge vital for implant stabilization and restoration of the 'posteromedial bulge'.

graft material that is of a sufficient size to be supported at its periphery on sound bone.

A large variety of materials have been advocated for the immediate repair of orbital floor defects. The list includes xenografts, allografts and autografts of fascia, bone and cartilage, and a number of resorbable and non-resorbable alloplastic materials. The latter, particularly titanium mesh and sheets of Silastic (medical grade silicone polymer), Medpor (porous polyethylene) and PDS (polydioxanone) have been widely used. Specially designed pre-shaped titanium mesh reconstruction plates with fixation flanges are also available and are

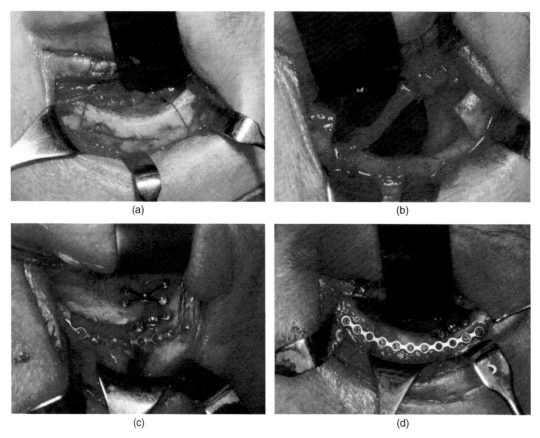

(a)   (b)

(c)   (d)

Figure 7.20 Inferior marginal orbitomy for improved visualization and access in repair of a large defect of the orbital floor. (a) Bone cuts made with fine saw. (b) Segment of rim removed with infraorbital nerve freed. (c) Repair of the defect, in this case with a calvarial bone graft. (d) Rim segment replaced and plated in position.

probably the best option currently available. They are particularly effective in recreating the anatomical shape of the orbital floor, a factor that is of key importance in restoring orbital volume and eye position (Fig. 7.21).

In view of reports of late complications with some alloplastic materials some surgeons prefer autogenous bone as a graft material. Resorption is minimized if dense cortical bone is used, for example from the outer table of the calvarium, but the bulk of the graft may be a problem in many defects. A useful source of thin autogenous bone is the anterior wall of the maxillary antrum that approximates to the curved shape of the orbital floor. Fixation of the implant or graft is not essential providing it sits passively and the periosteum can be sutured to prevent extrusion. If stabilization is required this can be performed by using microplates or by simple wiring to the orbital rim.

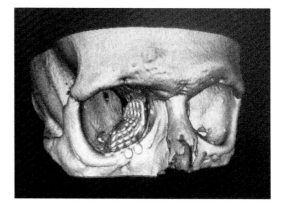

Figure 7.21 Three-dimensional CT scan showing a titanium mesh plate in place for reconstruction of the right orbital floor and medial wall.

The advent of CT scanning has revealed that associated medial wall fractures are quite common in orbital trauma. Often the defect is relatively small and does not contribute to the clinical problem. However, failure to address larger defects is likely to compromise the outcome following otherwise satisfactory orbital floor repair. Access to the medial orbital wall is possible through a number of approaches as described previously. It may be possible to explore the lower half of the wall through any of the standard infraorbital approaches, but access is somewhat limited and clear visualization of the entire wall can be very difficult. If this is required the transcaruncular extension of a transconjunctival incision gives excellent exposure. A coronal flap also provides good access to the upper half of the medial wall, and as such is very useful in the management of complex major trauma. However, it is an excessive approach for isolated medial wall defects.

Le Fort I, II and III fractures
General factors affecting treatment
There are a number of special anatomical problems in the midfacial region that complicate the basic principles of reduction and fixation in Le Fort type fractures. These are described next.

The complexity of the facial skeleton
Although the facial skeleton tends to fracture along broadly predictable lines of weakness, the resulting injury can be extremely complicated. It is very rare for the separated fragment to exist as a single block of bone. In the past the main guide for reduction of the fracture was the restoration of the occlusion and despite advances in internal fixation this still remains a crucial aspect of treatment in the dentate patient. However, because the mandible is moveable, simple re-establishment of the occlusion, for example by inter-maxillary fixation, only corrects the relative position of mandible to maxilla. This does not give a precise register of the position of the mobile midface in relation to the cranial base. Apart from restoration of the occlusion, the vertical and transverse dimensions of the midface need to be re-established in order to achieve the correct facial balance; the more complicated the fracture the more difficult this becomes.

Major midface injuries are often a complex of Le Fort I, II and III type fractures. Isolated Le Fort III fractures in particular are very rare. Furthermore, the nasal skeleton and the walls of the paranasal sinuses may be extensively comminuted and compressed into the main body of the skeleton of the midface. The restoration of facial form requires reconstruction of this complex facial shell, a task that is often hampered by the degree of comminution.

Other associated facial bone fractures
The fractured central midface is often only part of a complex that may include fractures of the mandible, zygoma, frontal bone and nose. Sometimes the inexperienced surgeon does not know where to start reorganizing these multiple displacements. This topic has previously been discussed in Chapter 1 (see p. 5) under 'Principles of treatment'. In summary, the outer ring or framework of the face is reconstructed first by reducing the frontal bone and orbital roof above, the zygomatic complex on each side and the mandibular platform below. Once the outer frame of the face is reformed the central block can be reduced and fixed within it, utilizing the occlusion as a locating point below and direct fixation to the reduced cranio-zygomatic complex as a key above. Finally, the nasal complex can be recontoured and supported in its correct relationship to the reduced central midfacial bone mass.

Airway management
The problems of reduction of the facial fractures are compounded by the need to maintain an airway and in most cases to administer a general anaesthetic. Under general anaesthesia it is usually difficult to re-establish the occlusion unless nasal intubation or tracheostomy is performed. Fortunately, nasendotracheal intubation, with fibreoptic guidance if required, is usually possible and low profile tubes can be positioned to lie laterally to allow surgical access to the whole facial skeleton. Tracheostomy should only be performed when there are specific surgical indications such as head or chest injury. Occasionally a reinforced oral endotracheal tube can be inserted to emerge through the mouth laterally posterior to the dentition in the retromolar region, and techniques have also been described in which the tube is brought out through a temporary surgically created passage through the floor of the mouth (submental intubation).

Problems of reduction and fixation
As noted previously, even if intermaxillary fixation is applied it is insufficient to reduce and stabilize the

middle third of the facial skeleton because of the mobility of the lower jaw. After using the mandible as a guide to accurate occlusal reduction, the middle third must be immobilized by attaching it to the adjacent facial bones. The complex methods of external fixation and internal wire suspension that were used in the past are now only of historical interest and, in common with mandibular fractures, open reduction and miniplate fixation is now the accepted treatment of choice for most midface fractures. Additional intermaxillary fixation is often advisable in complex trauma because gross comminution can make it difficult to obtain complete stability of the tooth bearing segment even if plates are used.

Surgical management
Reduction
Effective reduction of maxillary fractures depends primarily on thorough mobilization. The inherent degree of mobility of Le Fort fractures following injury varies considerably. To a large extent this depends on the amount of displacement and comminution. In some situations it may be possible to reduce low level maxillary fractures simply by finger manipulation alone. At the other extreme, with very firmly impacted Le Fort I and II fractures, it may be necessary to expose the fracture line through an incision in the buccal sulcus in order to mobilize it with an osteotome before reduction can be carried out.

The techniques described next, which were previously carried out for closed reduction of midface fractures, are still useful for mobilization and basic alignment of the fragments. They are a helpful preliminary step in the open reduction and plate fixation of Le Fort type fractures.

Le Fort I fractures (Guérin or low level fracture)
Rowe's disimpaction forceps are invaluable in the mobilization of most maxillary fractures. The maxilla is held with the paired forceps. Each unpadded blade is inserted into a nostril and the padded blade enters the mouth and grips the palate. Standing at the head of the operating table, the surgeon grasps the handles of each of the pairs of forceps and manipulates the fragments into place (Fig. 7.22). This is done by deliberate rocking and rotating movements in the sagittal and transverse planes, rather than simply attempting vigorous shaking in a misdirected manner.

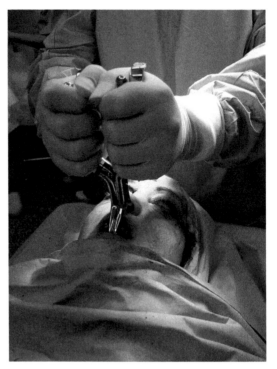

Figure 7.22 Rowe's disimpaction forceps in position for reduction of the tooth bearing portion of the upper jaw. (Reproduced with kind permission of Springer Science+Business Media.)

Forward traction can be applied once the fracture is mobile but significant posterior displacement is actually unusual in Le Fort I fractures. So-called lengthening of the face is a more common physical finding and special attention should be given to correcting any inferior displacement of the posterior aspect of the maxilla to relieve 'gagging' of the posterior teeth and a subsequent anterior open bite (apertognathia).

It is important to appreciate that some Le Fort I fractures may be in two or more segments with a mid-line split of the palate or a separate dentoalveolar fragment (Fig. 7.23). In this situation injudicious use of the Rowe's forceps can easily make matters worse and lead to an extensive laceration of the palatal mucosa.

Le Fort II fractures (pyramidal or sub-zygomatic fracture)
If the fracture is in one piece, it may be reduced in the same way as a Le Fort I fracture employing Rowe's disimpaction forceps. The fragment should be manipulated firmly away from the base of the skull until it is freely

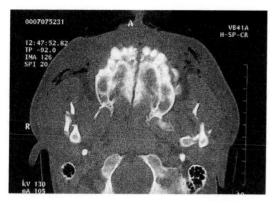

Figure 7.23 CT scan of patient with a low level fracture of the maxilla (Le Fort I type). A midline split of the palate is clearly demonstrated. In this situation any reduction using Rowe's forceps needs to be carried with extreme care to avoid further disruption of the fracture and tearing of the overlying mucosa.

mobile. It should not be shaken indiscriminately because the fracture line frequently involves the anterior cranial fossa that should not be further disrupted if at all possible. If, as is often the case, there is a coexisting Le Fort I fracture, manipulation with disimpaction forceps will only reduce the tooth-bearing portion. It may be difficult to mobilize the rest of the fragment without exposing the fracture but this can sometimes be effected by grasping the nasal septum with Asche's or Walsham's septal forceps, while at the same time inserting a finger of the other hand behind the soft palate and exerting forward pressure. If there is an associated naso-ethmoidal fracture this is treated after the tooth-bearing portion is adequately reduced and plated.

Le Fort III fractures (high level or supra-zygomatic fracture)

These severe injuries rarely occur in isolation but when they do, usually as a result of a lateral blow, displacement can be fairly minimal. More commonly, as a result of a frontal or oblique blow, there are associated Le Fort I and II fractures, often with separate zygomatic and nasal complex fractures. Extension of the fracture into the frontal bone and roof of the orbit may also occur (craniofacial fracture).

The structural pillars of the face are the key areas for assessment of the adequacy of reduction of complex facial fractures. It can be appreciated that the localization of the upper part of the midface depends on the frontal bone with its nasal and zygomatic processes,

whereas the lower part depends on the integrity of the zygomatic buttresses and the piriform aperture. These are also the areas most suitable for the application of bone plates. In the dentate patient occlusion with the intact mandible ensures accurate localization at the Le Fort I level.

Fixation

The current approach to internal fixation of Le Fort type fractures has resulted from developments in surgical technique shared with orthognathic and craniofacial surgery. The refinement of semi-rigid miniature bone plating systems has both accompanied and driven many of these developments.

Le Fort I fractures

Minimally displaced fractures of the edentulous maxilla may not need active treatment. In the dentate patient with a minimally displaced fracture that is not mobile three weeks of intermaxillary fixation is still an excellent and accurate method of treatment. The disadvantages of this time honoured approach have to be weighed against the technical problems of bone plating. This is an unforgiving technique that depends on anatomical reduction and completely passive adaptation of the plates if occlusal discrepancies are to be avoided.

Surgical exposure is achieved through a vestibular incision. Comminution of the anterolateral antral walls is common and small fragments may become detached as the periosteum is elevated. Reduction with Rowe's forceps, either before or after the exposure, can add further to this comminution. It is better to rely on temporary intermaxillary fixation to restore the occlusal relationship rather than simply offering up the mandible to the maxilla. Any displaced split of the palate should be reduced and repaired with a plate before applying the intermaxillary fixation and associated dentoalveolar fractures will require stabilization with an arch bar or splint.

Following the application of IMF the maxillo-mandibular complex is positioned passively prior to plating. It is important to ensure that the mandibular condyles are seated correctly in their fossae to prevent incorrect reduction and a subsequent anterior open bite. Inspection of the piriform aperture and zygomatic buttress areas will confirm the accuracy of the reduction and the fixation plates should then be applied. Even when there is comminution at the base of the zygomatic

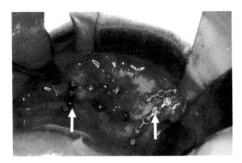

Figure 7.24 Operative view of internal fixation of the left side of a Le Fort I fracture. Comminution of the antral walls is a common feature of maxillary fractures and small fragments may become detached and lost. However, it is usually possible to plate the midface 'pillars' at the piriform aperture and base of the zygomatic buttress (arrowed).

buttress it is usually possible to find an area of bone contact between the alveolus and the buttress across which a plate can be placed, and similarly for the piriform area (Fig. 7.24).

At the end of the procedure the intermaxillary fixation is released and the occlusion is checked using passive movements of the mandible. Intermaxillary fixation is not necessary but may be desirable for a short period; particularly where there is comminution, a split palate, a separate dentoalveolar fracture, an associated mandibular fracture or where there is any doubt about the accuracy of the occlusal relationship.

Le Fort II fractures
Where the fracture is in a single block it can be treated in a similar manner to Le Fort I fractures. Plates are usually applied to the zygomatic buttress and infraorbital margin. Occasionally exposure can be sufficient using a vestibular incision, but usually the vestibular approach is supplemented by a lower eyelid or transconjunctival approach to the orbital rim. Alternatively a midfacial 'degloving' approach can be considered for more complex fractures if appropriate.

Le Fort II fractures are often associated with comminution of the nasal complex. A decision has to be taken as to whether the nasal fractures will be treated by closed reduction or whether open reduction and fixation is indicated.

Le Fort III fractures
As has been mentioned, monobloc Le Fort III fractures are exceedingly rare and are comparatively simple to treat by plating at the fronto-zygomatic and fronto-nasal sutures. More often the craniofacial disjunction is a combination of bilateral zygomatic complex, nasal complex and Le Fort II type fractures. This type of severe injury is also commonly associated with frontal bone fractures. CT scans will reveal the extent of fragmentation. Access to the whole upper and midface from the cranial base to the maxillary occlusal level is obtained by using a coronal scalp flap with an intra-oral vestibular incision. Additional bilateral approaches to the infraorbital rims and orbital floors are usually needed. This combination of incisions gives wide access for direct surgical repair of the upper and midface.

As has been stated previously the principle of management of these complex fractures is to reconstruct the outer facial frame first. This begins with fixation of both zygomatic complexes to the frontal bone laterally. Careful repair of a comminuted zygomatic arch is required to act as the basis for correct positioning of the main body of the zygoma (Fig. 7.7). If this is overlooked it may result in a failure to re-establish the forward projection and normal width of the bony midface (Fig. 7.25). There may be some rotation of the zygoma that can easily be missed. Since a coronal flap will almost certainly have been raised, it is technically easy and helpful to inspect the lateral wall of the orbit by retracting the anterior aspect of the temporalis muscle, and if necessary to apply a plate. Any rotation needs to be corrected prior to plating at the fronto-zygomatic suture.

Once the lateral orbito-zygomatic frame has been repaired attention is directed to the central midface block. The fractures are reduced and plates applied as necessary to the infraorbital rim and zygomatic buttress to rebuild the facial bones. Temporary intermaxillary fixation is used to locate the tooth bearing segment and to re-establish the occlusion with the mandible. Finally the nasal bones are manipulated and splinted.

Fractures of the naso-orbito-ethmoid complex

The naso-orbito-ethmoid complex (NOE complex) is formed by the skeleton of the nasal bridge and the bony structures between the orbits. Extensive fractures of this region are relatively uncommon but they present one of the most difficult challenges in facial trauma treatment. NOE fractures can present as an isolated injury following direct frontal trauma or as part of more complex extensive midface fractures. A unilateral or

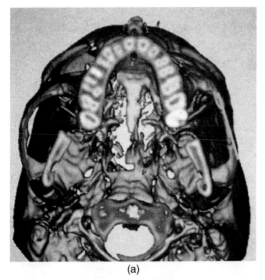

(a)

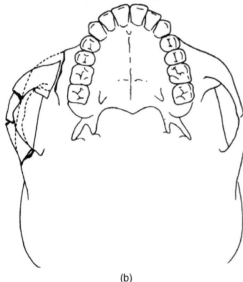

(b)

Figure 7.25 The significance of accurate zygomatic reduction for midface width and projection. (a) Posterior displacement of the zygomatic complex usually results in rounding of the arch (red) and loss of the normal straight profile (green). (b) Diagram showing how failure to correct this deformity in complex midface fractures will result in increased zygomatic width and postoperative flattening of the face.

bilateral pattern of fracture is possible. In essence the injury represents the most severe type of nasal fracture characterized by gross comminution of all the skeletal components, comprising to a greater or lesser extent the nasal bones, the frontal processes of the maxillae, the glabella, the lacrimal bones and the lamina papyracea of the ethmoid bones. The base of the nose is usually driven into the interorbital space with a characteristic upward displacement of the nasal tip and significant flattening of the nasal bridge.

Severe NOE trauma frequently disrupts the medial canthus. The medial canthal ligament is a condensation of fibrous tissue consisting of two limbs; a strong broad anterior limb attached to the anterior lacrimal crest and frontal process of the maxilla and a more poorly defined less important layer inserted into the posterior lacrimal crest. The lacrimal sac lies in the lacrimal fossa between the two limbs. The ligament acts as the tendon of origin of the orbicularis oculi and disruption of its attachment leads to loss of the normal acute angle of the medial aspect of the palpebral fissure. This results in a characteristic rounded appearance with an increase in the intercanthal distance (traumatic telecanthus).

The shape and normal relationship of the palpebral fissures is a most important cosmetic feature of the human face and even minor disturbance of this area causes a noticeable deformity (Fig. 7.26). If this goes uncorrected at the primary operation it is extremely difficult, if not impossible, to restore the appearance at a later stage.

Treatment

NOE fractures present a formidable reconstructive challenge if long term deformity is to be avoided. Effective treatment depends primarily on accurate replacement and fixation of the medial canthal ligaments and restoration of the nasal bridge anatomy. This is virtually impossible with closed reduction and external splinting, and the majority of cases will benefit from a more invasive strategy of open reduction and stable internal fixation. Despite this approach there are often difficulties in achieving and maintaining fracture reduction owing to the degree of comminution of the small thin bony fragments.

Closed reduction

This relies on manipulating the fragments into as good a position as possible and attempting to retain the reduction by splinting with acrylic buttons or small lead plates held in place with transnasal wires. The results are generally unsatisfactory because the wires and splints lie anterior to the anterior lacrimal crest and the insertion of the medial canthal ligament. It is difficult to prevent splaying of the moulding plates with

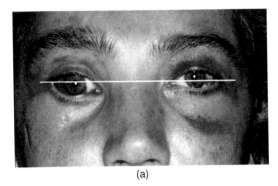

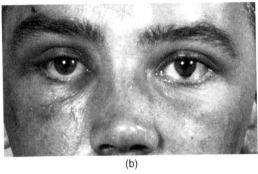

Figure 7.26 The importance of medial canthal anatomy. (a) NOE fracture with flattening of the nasal bridge and infero-lateral displacement of the right medial canthus. (b) Restoration of canthal position after open reduction and fixation using a coronal flap for access.

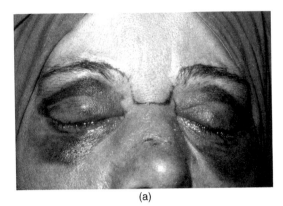

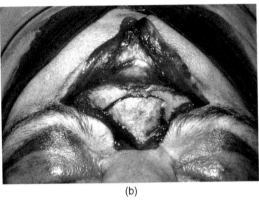

Figure 7.27 (a) Local incision used for exposure of a nasofrontal fracture. (b) Careful assessment of the injury is needed prior to using a local approach because the fracture may be found to be more complex than expected. A coronal flap is a safer option in most NOE fractures.

the result that collapse and flattening of the nasal base is virtually inevitable. Any vertical separation of the nasal and frontal bones will almost certainly go uncorrected. Secondary deformity is accordingly common after closed reduction; deformity that is difficult later to correct owing to scarring and displacement in the medial canthal area.

Open reduction and fixation

It is generally accepted that ORIF offers the best hope of restoring the anatomy of this area. Lacerations across the nasal bridge may occasionally be used for access and a number of local incisions have been described as mentioned earlier in the chapter. They all have the limitation of relatively restricted exposure (Fig 7.27). At operation the fractures may be found to extend into the adjacent frontal bones and midface, and any disruption of the medial orbital walls will also be difficult to manage.

The routine use of high resolution CT scans three-dimensional imaging in facial trauma has revealed the often complex nature and extent of these injuries and a coronal scalp flap should be the means of access in most cases. Wide subperiosteal dissection of the superior and lateral aspects of the orbits will facilitate exposure of the fronto-nasal region and the superior aspect of the medial orbital wall. Transconjunctival incisions with a lateral canthotomy (or other infraorbital approach) can be used in addition if exposure of the inferior aspect of the medial orbital wall and adjacent floor is needed.

The degree of comminution will influence the ease of dissection. This will be fairly straightforward over the stronger bone of the nasal bridge but care needs to be taken where the bone is thin and fragile in the region of the medial orbital wall and rim. A combination of standard subperiosteal stripping with a small elevator and sharp subperiosteal dissection with a scalpel will be required. The exposure should be sufficient to allow

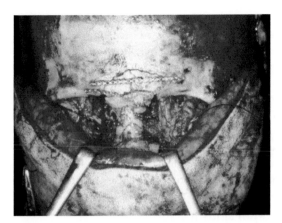

Figure 7.28 Open reduction and fixation of NOE fracture with frontal bone involvement. Wide exposure allows full assessment of the injury with the best possibility of restoring the complex anatomy.

accurate fixation whilst maintaining as much soft tissue attachment as possible to any small fragments of bone to minimize subsequent resorption. It is particularly important to identify any significant fragment still attached to the medial canthal ligament and to maintain this bony insertion.

The main objective of the reduction is to restore both the intercanthal distance; and the anterior projection and width of the nasal bridge. Where comminution is severe, or bone loss is evident, primary bone grafting may be required to achieve these ends.

Beginning with restoring an intact glabella, the nasal skeleton and medial orbital walls are rebuilt from above downwards (Fig. 7.28). The segment attached to the medial canthal ligament is carefully repositioned. The most common errors are under-correction of the inter-canthal distance and location of the repaired canthus too far anteriorly. A degree of overcorrection should be attempted and further support can be provided by external splinting once the incisions have been closed.

On rare occasions the canthal ligament may be avulsed from the bone, or the fragment may be too small to plate in position. In this situation a transnasal canthopexy should be carried out using fine wire or a braided stainless steel suture. Where the medial wall of the orbit is missing or extremely comminuted it is advisable to combine this with a bone graft or titanium mesh to help anchor the soft tissue (Fig. 7.29). Similarly, it may be better to consider a primary calvarial bone graft to the nasal bridge where extensive comminution is

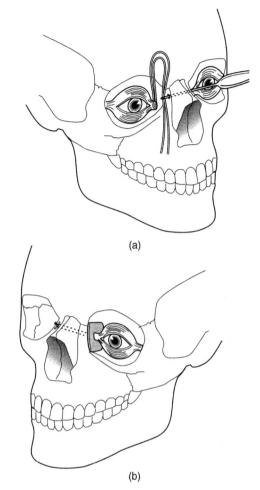

(a)

(b)

Figure 7.29 Diagram to illustrate the principle of transnasal canthopexy. (a) An awl or needle is passed through the nasal bones to pick up a braided wire suture attached to the canthal ligament. (b) The procedure may be combined with bone graft or titanium mesh reconstruction of the comminuted medial orbital wall. Even with these procedures post-traumatic canthal deformity is hard to prevent when the ligament has been completely detached.

present. This will help maintain the soft tissue envelope in a correct position and will minimize subsequent soft tissue contraction.

Management of nasolacrimal injuries

Despite its proximity to the naso-ethmoid region, the nasolacrimal system is damaged surprisingly rarely, even in severe maxillofacial injuries. The patency of the canaliculi and duct are difficult to assess at the time of presentation due to soft-tissue and mucosal oedema. It is more important to re-establish drainage through the lower canaliculus than the upper, and careful accurate repair of any soft-tissue lacerations in the area without any stent is the best way to facilitate this for the less-experienced surgeon.

Attempts to probe or irrigate the lacrimal system risk further damage, and exploration should be resisted unless there is obvious evidence of a transection due to laceration. If transection is detected the ends of a fine, soft silicone tube or nylon suture can be passed through the upper and lower lacrimal puncta to enter the nose, where they are tied together to lie beneath the inferior turbinate in the inferior meatus. This is not an easy procedure for the novice and if any difficulty is encountered in passing the stent the procedure should be abandoned before further damage is caused that will simply prejudice the outcome of any secondary corrective surgery.

If a stent is passed successfully the facial lacerations are repaired in the normal way and the stent is left in place for at least 3 months. Late obstructive symptoms following a facial fracture require appropriate investigation to isolate the site. This is usually within the bony nasolacrimal canal and is corrected by dacryocystorhinostomy.

Treatment of frontal sinus and craniofacial fractures

The frontal bone is the strongest part of the facial skeleton and fractures of the upper third of the face are therefore relatively uncommon. The anatomy of the frontal sinus has an important bearing on the management of frontal bone injuries. This varies from complete absence (4%) to extensive pneumatization that may even extend into the lesser wing of the sphenoid bone. In 10% of the population the sinus is unilateral. The frontal sinus has a thick strong anterior wall, a thin posterior wall and a fragile floor that also forms part of the roof of the orbit. There is usually a midline septum, and not uncommonly several other septa that partially subdivide the sinus cavity. Drainage of mucosal secretions is through the frontonasal duct that normally runs from the postero-medial aspect of the floor (nasofrontal recess) into the middle meatus. Like the sinus itself the duct anatomy is very variable. It can simply be a large foramen, or a true duct that extends from a few millimetres to up to 2 cm.

Many patients sustaining frontal and craniofacial trauma present with a closed head injury or other neurosurgical problems and will often require a combined operation with a neurosurgeon for optimal treatment. It is no longer considered essential to await full recovery from the brain injury prior to the definitive treatment of these fractures. Each case needs to be considered on its merits by an experienced neuro-anaesthetist but, generally speaking, if the prognosis for survival is considered good, combined relatively early repair by the maxillofacial and neurosurgical team may be possible.

Frontal sinus fractures

The management of frontal sinus fractures has been a matter of great debate. Part of the problem has been the relatively small number of patients studied and the length of time that can elapse before complications of treatment, or lack of treatment, will become evident. Furthermore, the patient may present some time later to a surgeon other than the one who treated the injury. For these and other reasons prospective randomized trials of various treatment alternatives are probably impossible. It is, however, accepted that the complications of delayed or improper treatment can be serious or even life threatening. They include cosmetic deformities, acute and chronic sinusitis, pneumocephalus, mucopyocoele, osteomyelitis, meningitis and brain abscess. Despite the potential seriousness of these complications it is still not known which particular fractures would inevitably result in such a problem if left untreated. Furthermore, even when treatment is deemed necessary, often because of neurosurgical concerns, there is still some lack of agreement on the most appropriate surgical option. What is generally agreed, however, is that the risk of late complications remains life-long.

Despite these comments some consensus is emerging with the recognition that a main aim of treatment should be to preserve a functioning sinus if at all possible, and to obliterate or cranialize it if it is not. A patent nasofrontal duct with unobstructed drainage is crucial for the maintenance of normal physiological function.

In summary the objectives of treatment are to create a 'safe sinus' and to restore the aesthetics. This may involve:

1 The elimination of any obvious factors predisposing to infection such as necrotic soft tissue or bone.

2 The preservation of normal sinus anatomy and function or, if this is not possible, the obliteration or cranialization of the sinus cavity.

3 The repair of any cosmetic defect.

Following frontal bone trauma the detection of cerebrospinal fluid rhinorrhoea is the most important clinical sign because it generally denotes posterior wall involvement. As with other maxillofacial fractures this may often settle with conservative management but if it is persistent neurosurgical intervention is almost certainly required. It has been noted previously that the key to normal sinus function is good drainage. It is essential therefore to assess possible damage to the frontonasal duct. High resolution CT scans, ideally including three-dimensional imaging, are mandatory to delineate the site and extent of the fractures.

There is no widely agreed classification of frontal sinus injuries. One simple classification divides fractures into those affecting the anterior wall only, those affecting both walls, and those affecting the posterior wall only. Isolated posterior wall fractures are rare but can occur in association with nasoethmoidal, orbital roof or other anterior cranial base fractures (Fig. 7.30).

Intervention in the past tended to be based too heavily on simply finding a fracture on CT resulting in a measure of over treatment. The degree of comminution and amount of displacement of the frontal bone fragments will in practice be of more importance as it is this that affects the patency or otherwise of the frontonasal duct. Accordingly, it is now recognized that accurate reduction of the fractures is the best way to restore the anatomy and hopefully a functioning duct. This may often be achieved without a craniotomy or 'radical' management of the sinus cavity although it will require clinical judgment and experience to decide the best option.

Anterior wall fracture

Approximately one third of frontal sinus fractures affect the anterior wall alone. Undisplaced fractures of the anterior wall do not need treatment unless firm fixation of the frontal bone is essential as a base for the repair of other naso-orbito-ethmoid or craniofacial fractures. More commonly there is displacement of the anterior table with an obvious visible or palpable forehead deformity. If there is no CT evidence of frontonasal duct involvement treatment should be concentrated on simply restoring the frontal contour. Occasionally an extensive laceration may give satisfactory access. For closed injuries, reduction using traction applied to screws inserted into the fragments through minimal forehead incisions has been described. There is increasing interest in endoscopic approaches to anterior frontal bone injuries, but this obviously requires experience in the use of this specialized equipment. In many situations it is safer to raise a coronal flap to allow good vision and a true assessment of the injury. Simple depressed fractures can be managed by elevation and fixation with low profile plates or bioresorbable mesh (Fig. 7.31). Compound injuries should be irrigated and cleaned, and any tissue with suspect vitality excised. If there are gaps in frontal contour due to bone loss in compound injuries these should be reconstructed with outer table calvarial grafts or titanium mesh.

Occasionally depressed frontal bone fractures can be safely left to heal and the residual cosmetic deformity dealt with using secondary onlay techniques.

With open repair it may be possible to inspect the sinus by removing a loose bone fragment. If so it is copiously irrigated and any contaminated or damaged mucosa excised. Otherwise the mucosa is left. The nasofrontal duct is inspected and if, as is usually the case, it is intact it is left alone. Drainage can sometimes be confirmed intraoperatively by instilling methylene blue or fluorescein into the sinus and detecting the dye in the nasal cavity.

Frontonasal duct involvement

It has been shown in animal experiments that obstruction of the frontonasal duct consistently leads to the production of a mucocoele. Radiographic assessment of duct injury is difficult even with the advent of CT

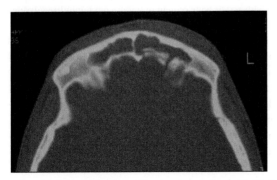

Figure 7.30 CT scan showing fracture of posterior wall of left frontal sinus with an intact anterior wall.

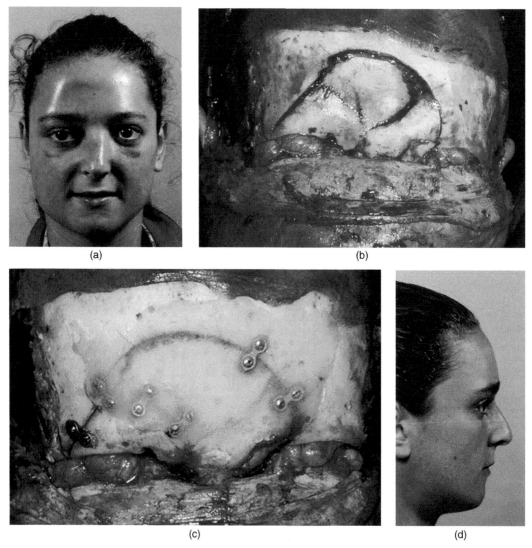

(a)   (b)

(c)   (d)

Figure 7.31 (a) Depressed fracture of frontal bone causing obvious cosmetic deformity of forehead. (b) Coronal flap raised to expose fractures. (c) Reduction and fixation. In this case the repair was covered with acrylic bone cement to smooth out minor irregularities and prevent plate palpation. (d) Lateral view showing post-operative appearance.

scans but should be suspected when there are associated naso-orbito-ethmoid or orbital roof fractures. Combined fractures of the anterior and posterior wall almost always extend into the posteromedial sinus floor to involve the duct but direct intraoperative inspection of the area is the best way to assess the situation.

If the posterior wall is intact treatment is directed at either re-establishing the drainage where possible or eliminating the sinus as a functional unit. Reduction of the fractures will help to restore the anatomy and this,

combined with removal of obviously damaged mucosa and opening of the nasofrontal recess, may well be all that is required. The midline septum can be removed as an additional safety measure to facilitate drainage from the uninjured side. Traditionally a silicone tube was placed and kept in place for several weeks but scarring and stenosis is common and secondary endoscopic techniques are more reliable if problems with drainage persist.

If it is clear at the time of surgery that the posterior wall is intact, but the duct is obviously badly disrupted and re-establishing drainage is very doubtful, then obliteration of the sinus is probably the safest option. This is a demanding procedure, particularly so in larger sinuses. It involves:

1 Complete stripping of the sinus mucosa, helped by the use of loupe magnification.
2 Removal of the cortical lining bone with a suitable bur to ensure complete elimination of the remnants of mucosa that are known to dip into small vascular pits on the bone surface.
3 Occlusion of the frontonasal duct with bone chips, muscle, or pericranium to prevent in-growth of mucosa from the nose.
4 Obliteration of the sinus cavity with either fat, muscle, bone chips, a pericranial flap, or biocompatible alloplast or bone cement.
5 Replacement of the anterior frontal bone segments.

Posterior wall fracture

The significance of posterior wall fractures is that they are associated with a high incidence of underlying dural tear with or without a demonstrable CSF leak. This is particularly likely in comminuted or displaced fractures. Conservative management can be considered in minimally displaced fractures but a persistent leak must be addressed to prevent infection.

Undisplaced or minimally displaced fractures with no indication for neurosurgical intervention can usually be managed as mentioned earlier for anterior wall injuries. However, displaced and comminuted fractures will require careful evaluation with combined neurosurgical and maxillofacial management. If intervention is indicated cranialization of the sinus is the method of choice to remove the risk of future intracranial infection. The principles of treatment are as follows:

1 A coronal scalp flap is raised with a large separate pericranial flap.
2 A frontal craniotomy is performed to expose the surface of the frontal lobes. Pre-drilling of holes for the miniplates will make replacement at the end of the procedure easier.
3 Loose fragments of anterior wall bone are carefully removed and kept in a suitable medium.
4 The posterior wall of the sinus is completely removed, as well as the inter-sinus septum and other septa.
5 Any intracranial injury is then treated and any dural tear repaired with a suitable graft.

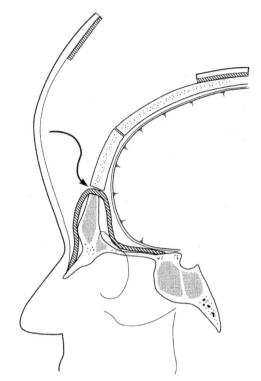

Figure 7.32 Diagram to show how a pericranial flap is used to reinforce the repair and separate the cranial cavity from the sinonasal cavity.

6 The sinus mucosa is stripped from the anterior wall bone and the inner cortex debrided as previously.
7 The frontonasal duct is occluded with bone dust or chips.
8 The pericranial flap is turned back to line the sinus floor and floor of the anterior cranial fossa. This key step gives additional protection to the exposed dura and ensures separation from the nasal cavity (Fig. 7.32).
9 Fractures of the anterior wall are repaired and the frontal craniotomy replaced and plated in position.

Combined craniofacial injuries

The management of the individual types of midface and upper face fractures have been discussed above. It has been noted throughout that the complex nature of the facial skeleton means that facial injuries often affect more than one bone. Where fractures of the frontal bone or cranium are associated with other fractures of the midface the term 'craniofacial fracture' is usually applied. These more severe injuries nearly always require joint neurosurgical assessment and treatment.

The various components are treated in sequence following the principles already discussed. The fronto-cranial fractures and intracranial injury are treated before treating the facial fractures. This will ensure that the superior aspect of the outer facial frame is established and will act as a guide for the midfacial repair, beginning with the zygomatic complexes. Fractures of the orbital roof may require bone grafting to prevent enophthalmos and orbital pulsation, particularly if they are comminuted. Posteriorly they can involve the optic nerves that may require intradural microsurgical decompression.

Further reading

Bell RB, Dierks EJ, Brar P, Potter. JK, Potter BE. A protocol for the management of frontal sinus fractures emphasizing sinus preservation. *J Oral Maxillofac Surg* 2007;65:825–839.

Burnstine MA. Clinical recommendations for repair of orbital facial fractures. *Curr Opin Ophthalmol.* 2003;14:236–240.

Chan J, Most SP. Diagnosis and management of nasal fractures. *Oper Tech Otolaryngol.* 2008;19:263–266.

Chang EL, Bernardino CR: Update on orbital trauma. *Curr Opin Ophthalmol.* 2004;15:411–415.

Cultrara A, Turk JB, Har-El G. Midfacial degloving approach for repair of naso-orbital-ethmoid and midfacial fractures. *Arch Facial Plast Surg.* 2004;6:133–135.

Ellis E., Zide MF. *Surgical Approaches to the Facial Skeleton.* 2nd Revised Edn. Lippincott Williams and Wilkins, 2005.

Herford AS, Ying T, Brown B. Outcomes of severely comminuted nasoorbitoethmoid fractures. *J Oral Maxillofac Surg.* 541 2005;63:1266–1277.

Manson PN, Clark N, Robertson B, Slezak S, Wheatly M, Vander Kolk C, Iliff N. Subunit principles in midface fractures: the importance of sagittal buttresses, soft-tissue reductions, and sequencing treatment of segmental fractures. *Plast Reconstr Surg.* 1999;103:1287–306.

Orlandi R, Knight J. Prolonged stenting of the frontal sinus. *Laryngoscope.* 2009;119:190–192.

Papadopoulos H, Salib NK. Management of naso-orbital-ethmoidal fractures [review]. *Oral Maxillofac Surg Clin North Am.* 2009;21:221–225.

Remmler D, Denny A, Gosain A, Subichin S. Role of three-dimensional computed tomography in the assessment of nasoorbitoethmoidal fractures. *Ann Plast Surg.* 2000;44:553–562; discussion 562–563.

Rohrich RJ, Adams Jr WP. Nasal fracture management: minimizing secondary nasal deformities. *Plast Reconstr Surg.* 2000;106: 266–273.

Schön R, Metzger MC, Zizelmannn C, Weyer N, Schmelzeisen R. Individually preformed titanium mesh implants for true-to-original repair of orbital fractures. *Int J Oral Maxillofac Surg.* 2006;35: 990–995.

Swinson BD, Jerjes W, Thompson G. Current practice in the management of frontal sinus fractures. *J Laryngol Otol.* 2004;118:927–932.

CHAPTER 8

Soft tissue injuries and fractures associated with tissue loss

Soft tissue injuries

'Soft tissues' is a non-specific term that can be interpreted to mean different things, but in the context of this book it refers to all the non-bony structures; including fat, muscle, nerves and blood vessels. In this respect it is important to remember it is more than just the skin. This is vital not only in the repair of soft tissue injuries but also in the planning of follow-up and aftercare. For example, the vascularity, and consequently the general health and quality of the soft tissue 'envelope', is a key element in gaining a satisfactory outcome in the management of all fractures.

Any wound that breaches the dermis will result in a permanent scar. How extensive this scarring is depends on a number of factors related to the type of trauma itself, the patient's biological makeup, the treatment received and the aftercare. Final outcomes, although partly beyond the operator's control, can still be greatly influenced by careful surgical technique and gentle handling of the tissues. Thorough wound toilet, judicious debridement and meticulous tissue handling are needed to achieve the best possible aesthetic and functional outcomes. Skin does not have the same protective mechanisms as the oral cavity (such as salivary growth factors) and infection may arise not only from external sources, but also from naturally occurring commensal organisms. This is more likely when there is devitalized tissue in the wound. Penetrating injuries need particular attention as bacteria are driven deep into the tissues where they are more difficult to eradicate.

Soft tissue facial injuries fall into three main groups:

1 Haematomas.
2 Simple lacerations.
3 Lacerations involving specialized structures or organs.

Haematomas

Most haematomas resolve over time, although occasionally they can fibrose, leaving a firm nodule in the soft tissues.

Auricular and nasal septal hematomas are important because of their potential to cause necrosis of the underlying cartilage. These require incision and drainage. The management of septal haematoma is described elsewhere (Chapter 7, p. 105). An auricular haematoma usually arises as a result of blunt trauma (Fig. 8.1). Following incision and drainage a compressive dressing is worn for several days. Failure to drain an auricular haematoma may result in a so-called 'cauliflower ear' as the haematoma undergoes fibrosis and contraction.

Very rarely haematomas in muscles can calcify, resulting in a disfiguring hard lump palpable under the skin. This traumatic myositis ossificans or heterotopic calcification is usually seen in the masseter muscle. Regular massage may help prevent this by breaking up the clot and any scar tissue that has formed.

Lacerations
Initial assessment

Always remember to examine carefully and document any tissue loss, ascertain the patient's tetanus status, and take a swab of contaminated wounds for microbiological culture. Broad spectrum antibiotics and tetanus prophylaxis should be prescribed according to local protocols.

Facial and scalp lacerations often bleed profusely. The management of bleeding has been described in Chapter 2. Once severe bleeding has been controlled sight threatening injuries always take precedence over other soft tissue damage.

The initial assessment of any laceration must take account of the factors that follow.

Fractures of the Facial Skeleton, Second Edition. Michael Perry, Andrew Brown and Peter Banks.
© 2015 John Wiley & Sons, Ltd. Published 2015 by John Wiley & Sons, Ltd.

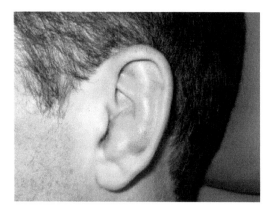

Figure 8.1 Haematoma of the left ear resulting in elevation of the skin overlying the concha and antihelix in particular. Drainage should be considered to prevent later deformity and possible necrosis of the cartilage. (Reproduced with kind permission of Springer Science+Business Media.)

Mechanism of injury

Sharp lacerations may be superficial or deep and in both the lips and eyelids, and may involve skin and mucosal surfaces as a 'through and through' laceration (Fig. 8.2). The condition of the skin edges is important. Shelving lacerations from windscreen glass are very difficult to repair with accurate edge approximation. Blunt trauma skin penetration may affect the vitality of the skin edges that may need to be judiciously trimmed before closure. All penetrating injuries carry bacteria into the deeper tissues.

Tissue loss

It is important to determine at an early stage whether there has been tissue loss. Initial appearances can often be deceptive: a blood clot may hold the wound together and disguise its extent, or retraction of skin flaps may create the appearance of tissue loss. The importance of tissue loss is anatomically related; loss of eyelid skin is more serious than the forehead or cheek, for example.

Contamination

The presence of very fine dirt particles within a laceration or abrasion will often lead to tattooing after healing even when the wound has apparently been thoroughly debrided prior to closure.

Foreign bodies

Foreign bodies within the tissues may range from fragments of glass or large dirt particles through to missiles

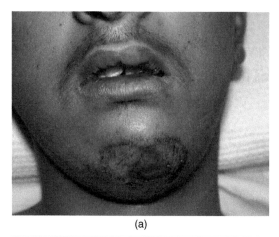

(a)

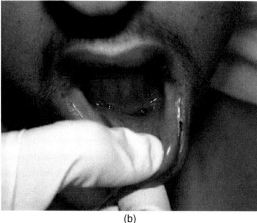

(b)

Figure 8.2 (a) 'Through and through' laceration of the chin. (b) What may appear on cursory examination to be a superficial injury actually extends through all layers to the oral cavity. Careful cleaning prior to repair is essential.

as small as airgun pellets or as large as bullets or shrapnel fragments.

Identifying foreign bodies within the tissues may require imaging. Plain films often suffice although CT may be needed to identify deeper objects and locate them more precisely. Magnetic Resonance Imaging (MRI) is obviously contraindicated in the presence of a metallic foreign body. If MRI is required to assess other head and neck injuries a plain radiograph or CT may need to be considered first to exclude any metal that may be present. MRI is useful in identifying non-metallic foreign bodies such as plastic but some materials, notably vegetation and wood fragments, may still be difficult to locate.

It should always be remembered that the final resting position of a projectile such as an air-gun pellet or bullet may be some way distant from the point of entry.

Injuries to underlying structures

The anatomy of the head and neck is such that even small lacerations may damage important structures. These include:

- Eye and lacrimal apparatus.
- Parotid duct and facial nerve.
- Sensory nerves.

Lacerations also frequently cross important anatomical boundaries such as the vermilion of the lip, the rim of the eyelid and the boundaries of the external nares. Precise alignment and closure is required, which may not be easily achieved by a non-specialist or inexperienced surgeon in the environment of a busy accident department. If there is any concern in this regard it is much better to refer the patient for management by a specialist.

Treatment logistics

Following initial assessment a number of logistical decisions need to be made some of which have already been mentioned. These include:

- When can the facial soft tissue be repaired taking account of possible other priorities in a multiple injury?
- Are other investigations such as imaging needed before a treatment plan can be agreed?
- Is there a need for consultation with other specialties, particularly ophthalmology?
- Does the definitive repair require special skills such as microsurgery for nerve transection?
- Is treatment possible or advisable under local analgesia?
- If treatment needs to be delayed what should be the intermediate wound care?

Facial wounds of special significance

There are a number of facial soft tissue injuries where repair should not be attempted by those without special training and knowledge. It is important that these are recognized so that appropriate referral can take place. Special consideration must be given to:

- Any wound with tissue loss. Gunshot wounds and other high velocity missile injuries in particular are rarely suitable for primary repair because of tissue necrosis and contamination. Delayed primary repair

after an intensive dressing regime is usually the treatment of choice (Fig. 8.3).

- Animal and human bites. The bacterial and saliva contamination of these injuries interferes with healing and repair may need to be modified.

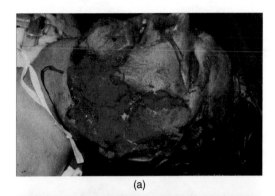

(a)

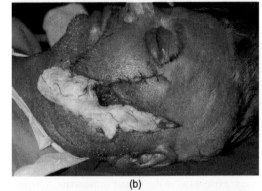

(b)

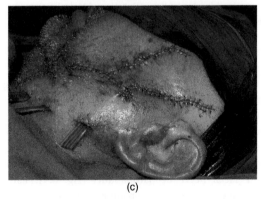

(c)

Figure 8.3 Contaminated shotgun wound to left face and jaw. (a) Following initial resuscitation, tracheostomy and packing of the wound. (b) Condition after several days of repeated lavage and wound dressing. A small area of tissue necrosis has become apparent. (c) Delayed primary closure and drainage. Despite initial appearances the final extent of tissue loss is minimal.

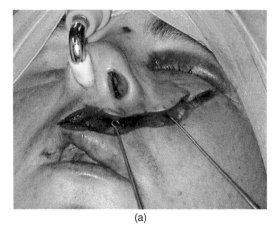

(a)

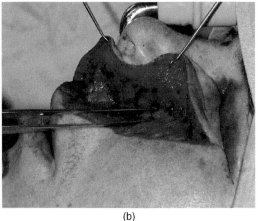

(b)

Figure 8.4 (a) Shelving laceration of upper lid and cheek. (b) Thorough exploration of the wound is important to retrieve any retained foreign bodies. (Courtesy of Malcolm Cameron, Addenbrooke's Hospital, Cambridge.)

- Shelved wounds such as those produced by glass fragments (Fig. 8.4).
- Lacerations of the eyelids particularly those involving the lacrimal canaliculi.
- Lip lacerations involving the red margin, where accurate realignment of both the muscle layer and the vermilion is critical.
- Cheek lacerations transecting major branches of the facial nerve or parotid duct (Fig. 8.5). Early microneural repair of the main branches of the facial nerve should be carried out.

Bites

Whether animal or human in origin, these must be considered as potentially serious injuries and managed

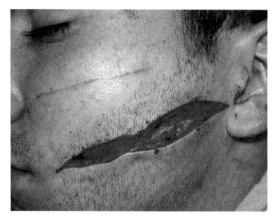

Figure 8.5 Knife wound to left cheek. Possible injuries to the facial nerve and parotid duct need to be identified in any laceration of this anatomical area. (Courtesy of Malcolm Cameron, Addenbrooke's Hospital, Cambridge.)

expeditiously. Both can rapidly become infected if they are not treated properly. Dog bites can range from simple puncture wounds, to irregular tears, to missing chunks of tissue. Canine teeth penetrate deeply, taking bacteria to the depth of the wound. Despite this, and unlike other sites on the body, bites and gashes on the face can often be closed primarily. However, they must be thoroughly cleaned and irrigated beforehand and should be monitored closely for signs of infection. All crushed and devitalized tissue should be carefully removed. More unusual bites, such as farmyard animals, snakes and so on, require specialist knowledge due to the risks of exotic infections or venom. Appropriate advice should always be sought.

Care of injured soft tissues prior to closure

Following arrest of haemorrhage careless handling of injured tissues prior to closure may compromise the outcome. This is especially so where primary closure has to be delayed either electively or due to the priority of other injuries.

Twisted or kinked flaps of tissue should be gently realigned and supported in their correct position as soon as possible. Loose sutures or adhesive paper strips should be used to hold them in place until definitive repair can be undertaken. Failure to do so may make the difference between an ischaemic but potentially salvageable soft tissue flap and a necrotic one. Owing to the excellent blood supply to the head and neck partially avulsed skin, even if attached by a small pedicle, may still have a good enough blood supply to enable it to heal if it is repositioned and secured.

If immediate closure of a facial laceration is not possible, the wound should be irrigated and covered with an appropriate dressing. If any delay beyond a few hours in definitive closure is anticipated, then gaping wounds in particular should be gently cleaned and loosely closed using adhesive paper strips or a few sutures and dressed.

Copious but gentle irrigation is the best way to clean a wound. Although a number of antiseptics are available some are reported to harm tissues and can delay healing. Sterile saline solution or water are not harmful to wounds and are generally recommended. Dirt contaminated wounds will require more vigorous cleaning as described in the following section. If antiseptics are used to clean or irrigate wounds care should be taken to protect the patient's eyes.

Definitive surgical management
Debridement and wound excision

Necrotic tissue can provide a focus for infection or lead to wound breakdown. Debridement may therefore be required. Wide excision is usually unnecessary on the face and is to be avoided if at all possible as this will result in a more extensive defect that will then be difficult to close primarily. This is particularly important around key sites such as the eyelids, nose and lips where any distortion of the tissues will result in significant functional and cosmetic problems. If an extensive area of soft tissue needs to be debrided an experienced opinion is needed at an early stage.

Tattooing can occur when grit and debris are not completely removed from a wound leaving visible particles under the healed skin surface. Foreign material must therefore be completely removed by meticulous wound cleaning and careful debridement. This may require prolonged but gentle scrubbing of the wound remembering that scrubbing in itself is additional trauma. Over-enthusiastic scrubbing can cause further damage to the wound and extend any zones of ischaemia. Small fibres from natural bristles can be left in the wound resulting in further foci for infection. If scrubbing is required use a small plastic brush, such as a soft toothbrush, and apply gentle pressure. Patience is needed since removal of all dirt particles may take some time. For small pieces of grit the tip of a pointed scalpel blade may be used to pick them from the wound.

Occasionally the wound edges may need to be minimally trimmed back to healthy bleeding tissue to achieve a clean closure but this is not needed in most facial lacerations and extreme care should be taken to avoid making the situation worse. Because of the excellent blood supply in the area the majority of facial lacerations heal satisfactorily and it is better to close the wound without any such interference. Scar revision can be considered later in the rare situation where it may be necessary. If wound contamination is extensive it is advisable to clean and debride as far as possible before dressing the wound and arranging for another wound inspection after 24–48 hours. Further debridement can be carried out at that stage if indicated before proceeding to definitive wound closure.

Primary closure of soft tissue injuries

Clean wounds should ideally be closed as soon as possible (within 12 hours) with accurate repositioning of the tissues. When suturing an irregular wound, look carefully for recognizable landmarks – matching these will greatly facilitate accurate closure (Fig. 8.6). If the wound edges are ragged, judicious trimming of the edges may convert an 'untidy' wound margin to a neat edge that can then be closed to give a superior aesthetic result. However, as already mentioned, this should be carried out with care and should be kept to an absolute minimum. Ideally there should be no tension across the wound but in cases where tension is a problem undermining of the skin, local flap closure, or skin grafts may rarely be used. If any doubt exists about viability of tissue it is better left in place and inspected later.

A good light and suitable instruments are essential and it is prudent to use an operating light rather than a less well-equipped clinic room. Deep lacerations are closed in layers with deeper tissues precisely aligned to eliminate any 'dead space' that would invite infection and compromises wound healing. When closing the skin the aim is to produce a neatly opposed and slightly everted wound edge. Inversion or stepping of the wound edges produces an inferior result and should be avoided. Sutures should not be tied too tightly; the correct tension being just short of that which causes localized blanching of the skin. Tight sutures will become tighter still with post-surgical swelling and may cut into the tissues leaving suture marks after healing with a cross hatched scar.

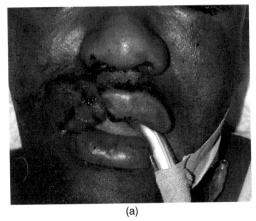

(a)

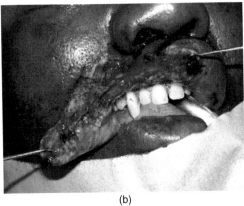

(b)

Figure 8.6 Full thickness laceration of upper lip involving the vermilion margin. (a) Wounds that involve key 'margins' (e.g. lip, nasal rim, ear or eyelid) require careful matching of anatomical landmarks. (b) In deep lip lacerations repair of the orbicularis muscle is also important. (Courtesy of Malcolm Cameron, Addenbrookes's Hospital, Cambridge.)

Alternatives to sutures include metal clips, adhesive paper tapes and skin adhesives such as cyanoacrylate glue. All these can be applied quickly but accurate alignment of skin edges can be difficult. Adhesive paper tapes and skin glues are especially useful in children and those who will not cooperate. The final cosmetic results are less predictable with these techniques compared with carefully placed sutures, largely because unsupported deep tissues may not be properly opposed.

Early removal of sutures (4–7 days) should be combined with continued support from an adhesive paper dressing or strips. This reduces the risk of wound dehiscence. Prolonged use of adhesive strips also helps reduce stretching of the immature scar.

Delayed closure and crushed tissues

Delayed closure may be unavoidable in patients with co-existing and more pressing injuries but usually results in poorer outcomes. Ideally thorough wound lavage and debridement should be undertaken as a preliminary stage, depending upon the degree of contamination and anticipated delay in definitive management. If there is a significant delay or the wound has been heavily contaminated wound drains may be used with advantage (see Fig. 8.3c).

Delayed primary closure may be necessary when doubt exists about the viability of a wound, or if it becomes infected. This is the likely situation following blast or high impact injuries. Crushed tissues are especially difficult to manage (Fig. 8.7). These may initially appear viable but later become necrotic. Multiple surgical procedures may be required. Split thickness skin grafts may be used as a temporary measure if there is tissue loss with revision surgery delayed until the patient has recovered or there are minimal risks of infection.

Healing by secondary intention

Healing by secondary intention is generally best avoided in the face and neck, as the aesthetic results are usually very poor. If primary closure or flap rotation into the defect is not possible, then skin grafts are often placed on

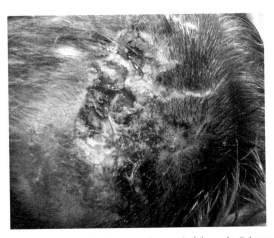

Figure 8.7 A crushed and contused wound of the scalp. Primary closure is not possible but a delay in treatment will allow any tissue of doubtful vitality to declare itself. With crush wounds healing by secondary intention or a skin graft may be indicated with revision surgery at a later date. (Perry (in press). Reproduced with kind permission of Springer Science + Business Media.)

Table 8.1 Stepwise options for the primary management of traumatic tissue loss.

---

1 Immediate replacement of avulsed tissue as a free graft.

2 Dress wound and allow to heal by secondary intention.

3 Direct closure under an acceptable degree of tension.

4 Partial or full thickness skin graft.

5 Immediate reconstruction with a free composite graft (e.g. some nasal defects).

6 Local or regional flap.

7 Avulsion of scalp/ear/nose: consider replantation using microsurgical techniques.

---

the wound bed to facilitate closure and minimize scarring. These are especially useful for small areas of tissue loss where local flaps will distort nearby structures.

Management of tissue loss

This is relatively uncommon but may be seen following gunshot injuries, industrial accidents and bites. More commonly, tissues are displaced rather than lost. Occasionally immediate replacement of the avulsed tissue (as a free graft) will result in a surprising degree of revascularization and healing although this is only possible with small volumes of clean tissue. This principle can be applied to partial loss of the nasal rim that can occasionally be successfully repaired using a graft taken from part of the pinna. Stepwise options for replacing lost tissue (sometimes referred to as the 'reconstructive ladder') are shown in Table 8.1.

Direct closure of a wound under some tension may succeed depending on the skins natural elasticity and ability to stretch or 'creep'. It is often an option in elderly patients where primary healing is more important than cosmesis. However, wounds closed under tension are more likely to break down with consequent distortion of nearby structures or a stretched scar.

Where a small amount of skin has been lost local flaps or skin grafts may be used to close or cover the defect. Full thickness skin grafts provide a better cosmetic result than split thickness grafts. To ensure the best possible colour match grafts should be harvested from the head and neck region (e.g. pre- and post-auricular, supraclavicular).

Skin flaps make use of the fact that there is often a small amount of excess skin on the face that is vascular and elastic enough to allow undermining and mobilizing to close adjacent defects. Numerous local flap designs

have been described in the literature and standard texts should be consulted for details of the techniques and indications. Local flaps are particularly useful in the reconstruction of nasal tips, eyelids and lips.

Major tissue loss is uncommon but may arise following industrial injuries, blast injuries or in pedestrians involved in motor vehicle collisions. Large defects such as scalp or ear avulsions are often a combination of soft and hard tissue loss. Whenever possible these patients should be considered for replantation. The avulsed tissue should be washed in sterile saline or water and sealed in a plastic bag. This bag should then be placed in a suitable refrigerator. For transportation, the sealed bag containing the avulsed tissue may be placed into a second bag containing a mixture of water and ice. It is important to avoid direct contact with ice that may further compromise vitality. In some cases it may be possible to replant the avulsed tissue and repair the arterial supply and venous outflow using microsurgical techniques.

Injuries to specialized tissues
Parotid injuries

Lacerations on the side of the face must be carefully assessed to exclude injuries to the parotid gland, parotid duct and most importantly the facial nerve. Injuries to the duct and nerve must be repaired before the skin is closed. Failure to repair the duct may result in the formation of a sialocele that will eventually drain percutaneously resulting in a persistent and often troublesome salivary fistula. Where possible the duct is repaired over a fine soft catheter stent.

Failure to repair the facial nerve results in a varying amount of facial weakness. As a 'rule of thumb' if facial weakness results from a laceration antero-medial to a vertical line dropped perpendicularly from the lateral canthus the nerve branches are usually regarded as too small to repair. Postero-lateral to this line the cut nerve should be identified and repaired if possible. Ideally repair should be undertaken as soon as possible, and no later than 72 hours after injury, unless the wound is heavily contaminated. If direct suturing of the divided ends is not possible an interpositional nerve graft may be necessary.

Eyelid lacerations

Soft tissue injuries of the periorbital region usually demand specialist care from the outset. Examination

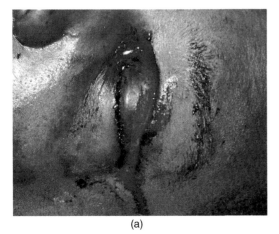

(a)

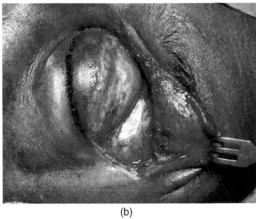

(b)

Figure 8.8 (a) Shelving upper eyelid laceration. (b) Although quite deep with exposure of the orbital rim, repair was uncomplicated because the lid margin and the levator apparatus were not involved. Specialist referral is indicated for management of complex lid injuries. (Courtesy of Malcolm Cameron, Addenbrooke's Hospital, Cambridge.)

under anaesthesia may be necessary to assess the wound completely and establish priorities. Assessment and management of any associated ocular injury is more important than that of the eyelid and has been described in Chapter 2.

Only simple eyelid lacerations should be repaired under local anaesthesia (Fig. 8.8). Superficial cuts can often be aligned and taped with no sutures. It is important that any suture ends do not rub the cornea and cause abrasions. Complex lacerations such as those involving the lid margin, canthal regions, medial third of the lids and levator muscle must be referred to a specialist for an opinion. These lacerations can disrupt

the lacrimal drainage system and functional integrity of the lid and thus require detailed understanding of the functional and aesthetic anatomy of the region. No tissue should be excised. The eyelids have an excellent blood supply and even quite necrotic-looking tissue can often survive.

Fractures associated with tissue loss

Although this type of major injury can occur as a result of certain industrial injuries or by fast-moving objects, it is more commonly associated with missiles employed in war or violent civil disturbance. In recent years civil unrest has frequently involved the use of firearms and the general severity of facial injuries resulting from urban violence has increased throughout the world such that there has been a blurring of civilian and military injuries. Firearm injury in the United States averaged 32,300 deaths annually between 1980 and 2007 and is the second leading cause of injury death after motor vehicle accidents. The main differences between fractures due to missile injuries and those resulting from blunt trauma can be enumerated as follows:

1 Fractures are usually extensively comminuted.
2 Fractures are always compound and the wounds contaminated by foreign matter and bacteria.
3 The viability of the bone fragments and the extent of injury to teeth cannot be accurately evaluated preoperatively from clinical and radiographic examination.
4 Wound treatment and the management of any underlying fracture is complicated by actual or potential composite tissue loss (Fig. 8.9).

Factors affecting the wounding capacity of missiles
Energy transfer
Bullets and other missiles travelling at high velocities have the capacity to produce extensive damage because of the release of kinetic energy at the point of impact. Kinetic energy is proportional to the square of the velocity ($E = \frac{1}{2}mv^2$) and it is therefore the impact velocity of the missile that is the most important factor. At impact there is deformation and sometimes fragmentation of the missile. The release of energy during passage through tissues produces temporary cavitation and tissue may be devitalized beyond the visible track of

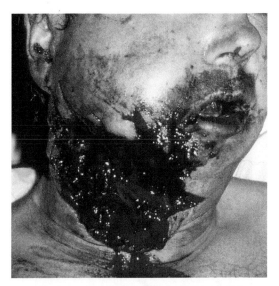

Figure 8.9 Missile injury to right face, neck and mandible. Gross comminution, wound contamination and a variable amount of tissue loss are features of this type of injury.

the missile. These factors result in widespread damage adjacent to the missile tract and an 'explosive' exit wound, although the entry wound may be comparatively small. The energy transfer from a missile at the point of impact is affected by the shape of the missile and the tissue density as well as the impact velocity. Missile wounds are generally classified as resulting from either 'high energy' or 'low energy' transfer.

Type of Missile
Bullets
In general hand-gun bullets are larger than rifle bullets and are fired at lower velocity. The casing of rifle bullets is important because it is designed to prevent fragmentation of the bullet. Soft-nosed rifle bullets expand on impact and cause more extensive tissue destruction than military bullets.

Fragments
Fragmentation missiles are more common than bullets as a cause of injury in modern warfare. Fragments originate from shells, mines, bombs and grenades of various designs. Such primary fragments can be irregular or, as in the contents of grenades, preformed. In addition, wounds can occur from secondary fragments arising from the general environment; debris from destroyed buildings for instance.

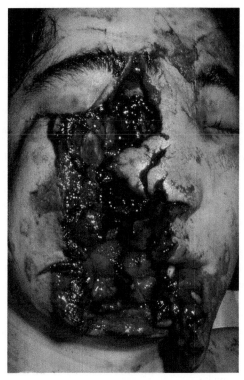

Figure 8.10 Shotgun injury resulting from an unsuccessful suicide attempt. Note the heavy contamination of soft tissues with fragmentation and partial loss of both anterior mandible and maxilla. Even though shotgun cartridges are fired at a relatively low velocity this is sufficient at close range, combined with the heavy mass, to result in a 'high energy transfer' injury.

Shotgun ammunition
Shotgun cartridges are quite different from bullets. They are designed to generate a spread of shot over a short range at relatively low velocity. Fired at short range as in a suicide attempt, they can produce massive tissue damage (Fig. 8.10). This is because the actual charge is a heavy load of metal backed by other packing materials such as felt. If fired at a range of less than 3 metres this charge remains compact and is of sufficient mass and velocity to result in a high energy transfer injury.

Physical properties of target tissue
In general the higher the tissue density the higher the energy transfer on impact. If a missile is stopped virtually completely by impact with bone all the available energy is instantly released. The effect on less resistant tissues is not so clear cut and damage is greatly influenced by the actual behaviour of the missile within the tissues.

Missile behaviour within tissue

The important features of missile behaviour are either fragmentation within the tissues or the effects resulting from deviation of a bullet from its true path (yaw and tumble). In either case tissue damage is increased. For instance deformation of unjacketed low velocity lead bullets is high, but the damage is confined to the path of the bullet. Conversely, soft nosed bullets from high velocity sporting rifles mushroom on contact that in turn stops the bullet resulting in high energy transfer with maximum tissue damage – ideal for stopping an elephant charging but regarded as immoral in warfare. Bullets from smaller high velocity modern rifles (muzzle velocity >900 m/sec) exhibit extreme amounts of yaw, and also fragment within the tissues, resulting in a larger exit than entry wound.

Missile fragments are mostly non-aerodynamic, with the exception of flechettes. However, they may be large and of very high velocity at short range with devastating energy transfer. The physical size of a primary or secondary fragment may result in a low degree of penetration but they produce an extreme degree of laceration and crushing. Multiple wounds are common from shells and grenades.

Effects of clothing and body armour

Penetrating missiles carry particles of clothing and any protective body armour into the wound, although this is generally less relevant in the facial region. Dirty contaminated clothing has been an important factor in wound contamination in many historical conflicts.

Principles of treatment

It can be seen that the biophysical factors enumerated above mean that wounds of similar appearance on the surface are associated with varying degrees of internal damage. It is important therefore to 'treat the wound rather than the weapon'. Tissue loss may be apparent or potential and such injuries often require protracted treatment. Management can be divided into four main phases.

Immediate post-traumatic phase

The patient is not particularly shocked as a result of a facial injury alone but haemorrhage may be severe. These patients are often fully conscious even after extensive injury and maintain surprisingly good control over their own airway as they are able to position

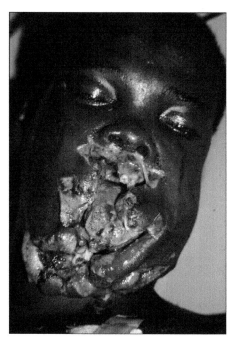

Figure 8.11 War injury resulting from a missile fragment. The patient maintained consciousness unaided and survived 4 days in transit from a remote area to a maxillofacial unit without any medical help apart from a battlefield dressing.

themselves so that blood and debris do not obstruct respiration (Fig. 8.11). Care must be taken in transporting such patients to ensure they are not laid on their backs in which position they may rapidly suffocate. They should be laid face downward with their head supported clear of the end of the stretcher, or lying on their side in the 'recovery position'. Either position ensures that the tongue falls forward and blood and saliva drain out of the mouth. Ambulatory patients will spontaneously hold their face downward and forward. If the injured person is unconscious, or consciousness is depressed, immediate steps must be taken to remove blood and debris from the mouth and to control the tongue by a traction suture if necessary. Consideration may have to be given to the establishment of an emergency airway at the scene but once medical facilities are reached ATLS principles can be applied and the patient intubated.

These patients suffer surprisingly little pain considering the extent of the injury and powerful analgesics that depress the cough reflex should not be administered unless an airway has been secured.

Primary surgical phase

Extensive wounds usually require a tracheostomy to ensure immediate and ongoing postoperative control of the airway. Assessment of tissue loss as opposed to tissue damage is very important in the initial evaluation. The surgical treatment of the fractures is often an incidental stage in the management of the wound as a whole. The basic stages of treatment can be summarized as follows:

Wound toilet

A missile injury is always contaminated and intensive preliminary toilet is necessary in most cases, before any formal surgical closure is considered.

Debridement

When the wound is ready for definitive surgery thorough debridement should be carried out to remove all devitalized tissue. In many cases a suitable period of observation is advisable to allow necrotic tissue to declare itself and serial debridement may be required in very high energy injuries.

Management of involved teeth

Teeth are both a source of subsequent wound infection and a possible means of intermaxillary fixation (IMF). Their status in these two respects may only be determined by inspection at the time of primary surgery. It is therefore very difficult to determine the method of fixation with any confidence before the patient is under an anaesthetic. In general all extensively damaged and subluxed teeth should be removed. There are, however, occasions when temporary retention of damaged teeth may be necessary simply to control large loose alveolar fragments. Infection and delayed healing may result from such a decision in which case the involved teeth are removed at a later date by which time some consolidation of the bone fragments will have occurred.

Reduction and fixation

In mandibular fractures every attempt must be made to establish bone continuity especially in the symphysis region. This can sometimes be achieved by deliberately displacing fragments to compensate for small amounts of bone loss. Where irretrievable significant bone loss has taken place the remaining portions of the mandible should be positioned in their normal relationship and separately immobilized. Options include internal rigid fixation, external fixation or IMF. The relative merits of

these are discussed in the chapter on mandibular fractures (Chapter 5).

Missile injuries to the mid-facial region rarely cause complete separation of bone from the skull base as in classical Le Fort type fractures. They do, however, cause considerable local comminution and loss of bone, loss of soft tissue and penetrating injuries of the orbit, paranasal sinuses and sometimes the cranial cavity. Overall wound management is more important than fracture reduction apart from dentoalveolar injuries.

Closure of mucosa and skin

The oral mucosa is closed first after underlying fractures have been suitably reduced and stabilized. Every attempt should be made to ensure that this closure is watertight. Because of the degree of comminution and bone loss, IMF is often needed as an adjunct to internal or external fixation. Once the jaws are immobilized the overlying skin wound is repaired. The degree of skin loss is often less than it first appears, but when it has occurred it is often possible to obtain closure by undermining the wound edges or by raising local or regional flaps. The historical technique of skin to mucosa suturing should only be used as a last resort as it condemns the patient to extensive secondary reconstruction. Every effort must be made to reconstitute the oral sphincter at an early stage even if this results in some distortion or reduction in size of the mouth orifice.

Drainage

Comminuted bone within a sleeve of healthy periosteum will heal in continuity. If, however, the periosteal sleeve becomes infected the fragments of bone will necrose and sequestrate leading to non-union. For this reason drains should be used liberally in contaminated comminuted fractures of the mandible. Through-and-through drains that allow subsequent irrigation of the fracture site are often helpful in preventing or controlling infection. It must be remembered that all missile wounds are infected from the outset, however 'clean' they may appear after initial debridement.

Immediate postoperative phase

Patients who have sustained severe facial injuries of this nature are very conscious of their actual and potential deformity. They require sympathetic nursing and psychological support. Special feeding devices or enteral feeding tubes may be needed if there is soft tissue loss involving the oral sphincter and sometimes some form of saliva shield may have to be constructed to prevent the constant escape of oral secretions. Oral hygiene is, of course, even more important than in simpler fractures and patients usually require active assistance with mouth irrigation and cleaning.

Reconstructive phase

There is no doubt that surgical expertise in treating the original injury can do much to reduce the amount of later reconstruction. If mandibular continuity is established, even with considerable loss of mandibular thickness, function is restored more quickly and the need for later bone grafting minimized. Similarly, ingenuity in the use of local flaps during initial wound closure will minimize the effects of skin loss.

Nevertheless some secondary reconstruction is usually necessary. Skin may have to be brought in and bone contour modified or re-established. Teeth need to be replaced and many patients require special prostheses. The reconstructive phase of treatment of these extensive disfiguring injuries may involve numerous hospital visits and further operations over a considerable period of time. If free tissue transfer with microvascular anastomosis is envisaged at any stage it is important to appreciate that endovascular damage to surrounding blood vessels may have occurred due to the energy transfer at the time of injury.

Further reading

Allonby-Neve CL, Okereke CD. Current management of facial wounds in UK accident and emergency departments. *Ann R Coll Surg Engl.* 2006;88:144–150.

Baker SR. (ed.) *Local Flaps in Facial Reconstruction.* 3rd Edn. Elsevier Saunders, 2014.

Hogg NJ, Horswell BB. Soft tissue pediatric facial trauma: a review. *J Can Dent Assoc.* 2006;72:549–552.

Lisman R, Spinelli H. Orbital adenexal injuries. In: *Surgery with Facial Bone Fractures.* Sherman JE, (ed.). New York: Churchill Livingstone; 1987:108.

Nicks BA, Ayello EA, Woo K, Nitzki-George D, Sibbald RG. Acute wound management: revisiting the approach to assessment, irrigation, and closure considerations. *Int J Emerg Med.* 2010;3:399–407.

Patel KG, Sykes JM. Management of soft-tissue trauma to the face. *Operative Tech Otolaryngol-Head Neck Surg.* 2008;19:90–97.

Sadda RS. Maxillofacial war injuries during the Iraq-Iran war. *Int J Oral Maxillofac Surg.* 2003;32;209–214

Ueeck BA. Penetrating injuries to the face: Delayed versus primary treatment – considerations for delayed treatment. *J Oral Maxillofac Surg.* 2007;65:1209–1214.

CHAPTER 9

Postoperative care

In contrast to the assessment, management and complications of facial injuries, comparatively little has been published specifically addressing the follow-up process in trauma and the particulars of aftercare. Postoperative care protocols vary considerably and are often based on individual opinion, rather than any rigorous evidence base. Patients may be followed up for only a month or two, or may be kept under review for a number of years depending on the surgeon's interest, the development of ongoing complications and the need for further surgery. Financial and other constraints may also influence the decision to discharge patients. Yet it could be argued that extended follow up is important for the assessment and publication of long-term outcomes necessary for good 'quality control' in trauma. Lack of complications alone does not necessarily define a good outcome. Nevertheless, a pragmatic approach is usually required in practice, particularly in centres where high volumes of trauma and limited resources make it impossible to provide long term follow up for every patient. In addition many trauma patients, if they are asymptomatic or have no obvious concerns, are understandably reluctant to continue to keep clinical review appointments. As well as the points mentioned previously, there are a number of general factors that should be taken into account when planning the review of a facial trauma patient, as listed in Table 9.1.

The surgical treatment of injuries associated with the patient's airway gives rise to special postoperative problems. Those problems are compounded if the jaws have to be immobilized before the patient has fully regained conscious control of the airway. The advent of direct osteosynthesis has made postoperative care simpler and safer as prolonged intermaxillary fixation (IMF) for fractures involving the dentition has become an infrequent requirement. Whenever possible, treatment should be designed to avoid IMF during the period of recovery from anaesthesia even if it will be applied electively once the patient is fully conscious.

Postoperative care may be divided into three phases:

1 The immediate postoperative phase when the patient is recovering from the general anaesthetic.
2 The intermediate phase before clinical bony union has become established.
3 The late postoperative phase that includes removal of fixation, occlusal rehabilitation, physiotherapy and long-term review of dental health in particular.

Immediate postoperative care

General care

Most maxillofacial units have access to a post-surgical recovery unit, surgical high dependency unit or intensive care unit to which patients can be transferred from the operating room and where they can be kept under skilled nursing supervision until they are fully recovered from the anaesthetic and fit to be transferred back to their ward. In the absence of such facilities an experienced nurse should remain with the patient until recovery is complete.

Some facial injuries may be associated with other critical injuries. During the postoperative period these patients will require monitoring in a high dependency or intensive care unit until they are fully conscious and systemically stable (Table 9.2).

Care of the maxillofacial injury

Ideally patients should be returned from the operating room with a nasopharyngeal airway in position, particularly if there is concern about swelling or continued oozing of post-nasal or intraoral blood. This should be left *in situ* until the patient recovers consciousness. They should be nursed lying on their side during recovery to

Fractures of the Facial Skeleton, Second Edition. Michael Perry, Andrew Brown and Peter Banks.
© 2015 John Wiley & Sons, Ltd. Published 2015 by John Wiley & Sons, Ltd.

Table 9.1 Clinical factors to be considered in the review plan for a facial trauma patient.

1 Most fractures are healed sufficiently to support functional loads (notably biting or chewing) by about one month. Comminuted fractures will probably take a little longer.
2 Residual enophthalmos will usually be apparent by about three months, if not sooner.
3 Minor residual diplopia can take many months to resolve (if at all).
4 Plates and screws can become infected within days, but may take years. (Smokers are especially at risk.)
5 Soft tissue injuries and scars can take 18 months or longer to mature enough to give an indication of the final result.
6 Lymphoedema can take many months to settle, particularly around the eyelids.
7 Nerve injuries can take 18 months or longer to recover.
8 Mucocoele formation (notably frontal sinus and lacrimal) can take several years to become clinically apparent.
9 Some authorities believe the risk of meningitis following inadequate management of the frontal sinus is life-long.
10 Condylar resorption can take years to become clinically apparent.
11 Dental or periodontal complications can take many months or even years to become clinically apparent.
12 Post-traumatic psychological complications can last a lifetime.

Table 9.2 Essential elements of care for the high dependency patient.

1 Control of the airway, including tracheostomy care if needed.
2 Monitoring the level of consciousness.
3 Detection of circulatory failure from clinical observations (pulse, blood pressure, urine output, central venous pressure).
4 Detection of respiratory difficulties from clinical observations (respiratory rate, oxygen saturation).
5 Monitoring possible abdominal changes (bowel sounds, urine output, distension, tenderness).
6 Prevention of sepsis, stress ulceration and venous thromboembolism.
7 Maintenance of hydration and nutrition.

enable any saliva or oozing blood to escape from the mouth. Good lighting and efficient suction apparatus to which a flexible suction catheter is attached must be at the patient's bedside. This enables the nurse or carer to pass the tube down the nasopharyngeal airway or nasal passages to suck out the nasopharynx. The suction tube can also be passed along the buccal sulcus to keep this area free of secretions. A rigid pharyngeal sucker should

also be to hand for more efficient emergency intervention if required.

Although IMF can usually be avoided in the immediate postoperative period there are still some situations where this traditional method of treatment may have to be employed. In such cases instruments such as scissors and wire cutters must be available at the patient's bedside so that the fixation can be released in an emergency. Physical control of the tongue with a traction suture in a recovering patient may be indicated if there has been extensive soft-tissue injury to the oropharynx or in a patient whose level of consciousness is expected to remain depressed after initial recovery. However, patients in this category will normally remain on assisted ventilation via either an elective tracheostomy or prolonged endotracheal intubation.

Postoperative vomiting should not be a problem if the patient has been correctly prepared for operation. If a genuine emergency operation is required, there may be significant amounts of recently swallowed blood as well as food within the stomach. In these circumstances it may be necessary to evacuate the stomach contents before anaesthetizing the patient. Modern anaesthetic techniques have reduced the incidence of postoperative vomiting to negligible proportions. Should it occur, although extremely unpleasant for the patient, vomiting whilst in IMF does not usually represent a danger to the airway providing full consciousness has been regained. Any liquid stomach contents can be expelled through closed teeth aided by suction in the buccal sulci.

Fractures of the midface often involve the orbit and, if this is the case, it is essential that vision and visual acuity are assessed at the earliest opportunity. An examination should be made and recorded as soon as the patient is conscious and regular checks need to be made during the first few hours after surgery. Fractures of the zygomatic complex must be protected from displacement during this period particularly when direct osteosynthesis has not been used.

If for any reason the Glasgow Coma Score was being recorded immediately pre-operatively (see Appendix to Chapter 2) this should obviously continue. Checks should be made for CSF leaks in patients with high level midface and craniofacial fractures.

Although very rarely used in modern practice, any patient with external pin fixation needs careful nursing if restless during recovery to avoid damage to the apparatus.

Intermediate postoperative care

General supervision

Patients who have sustained a maxillofacial injury will rarely require high dependency care after the first postoperative 24 hours. After this they should be carefully examined at regular ward rounds. Initial checks focus on the temperature, pulse and blood pressure and, when necessary, fluid balance and pain control. Prescribed drugs should be reviewed. In all patients the occlusion should be checked as early as possible. Direct osteosynthesis carries with it a risk of malalignment unless very carefully applied. Unacceptable reduction needs to be corrected at an early stage, by further surgery if necessary. Intermaxillary fixation, if in place, must be inspected to ensure the postoperative reduction has been maintained and fixation has not become loose.

Reduced midfacial fractures should be carefully examined to ensure the contour of the face has been restored. This is particularly important for high level Le Fort type and zygomatic complex fractures. Eye movements must be checked and diplopia or reduced visual acuity noted, regularly reviewed and urgently referred if necessary. Simple assessment of diplopia by following the examiner's finger should be tested a full arm's length in front of the patient and examination of visual acuity must take account of any eye ointment or fluid, which may affect light perception.

The alignment of the nasal skeleton must be assessed clinically and any persistent or new CSF leakage noted. Nasal secretions can be troublesome for the patient and a 'bolster' dressing across the external nares to absorb these is helpful in the early postoperative period. It will require regular replacement for patient comfort.

All these clinical observations should be supported by early postoperative radiographs, often including CT in complex cases, to confirm that satisfactory reduction and fixation has been achieved.

Adequately reduced and immobilized facial bone fractures are relatively painless and the postoperative oedema rapidly subsides. Light cold compresses applied to areas of swelling may help relieve discomfort and reduce swelling. Proprietary devices irrigated with cold saline that are specifically made for this purpose are now available. Any increase in swelling, particularly if accompanied by signs of active infection, requires immediate attention.

Posture

Patients with a fracture of the facial skeleton find it more comfortable if they are in the sitting position with the chin well forward. Providing there is no contraindication to this posture the conscious patient should be nursed in this position. The unconscious ventilated patient obviously does not require postural assistance of this nature but will need repeated mouth toilet and suction to remove accumulated blood and secretions.

Sedation

If the fracture has been adequately reduced and effectively immobilized, the patient should experience very little significant pain so that large amounts of postoperative analgesics are seldom indicated and should not be administered routinely.

Opiates should be avoided if possible in patients with maxillofacial injuries. These drugs depress the respiratory centre and cough reflex and for these reasons alone they are potentially dangerous if given to patients who may already have compromised airway function due to postoperative swelling or IMF. The use of any powerful analgesic may mask a deteriorating level of consciousness and morphine derivatives cause constriction of the pupil that obscures the pupillary changes indicative of a rise in intracranial pressure. Patients with maxillofacial trauma may have sustained injuries elsewhere and it is important that the physical signs of, for example, a compartment syndrome are not unnecessarily suppressed by potent analgesics. It should always be remembered that restlessness in a recovering patient may be due to airway difficulties but other sources of discomfort such as a distended bladder must not be overlooked.

Patients who are cerebrally irritated will remain in the intensive care environment with sufficient sedation to allow assisted ventilation through a secure airway.

Prevention of infection

Cleaned and sutured facial lacerations, with the exception of animal bites and heavily contaminated wounds, do not require prophylactic antibiotics. The same can be said of all closed fractures of the facial skeleton such as the zygomatic complex and edentulous parts of the mandible or maxilla. However, fractures of the tooth-bearing areas are more liable to infection and prophylactic antibiotics are usually given. Unless contraindicated penicillin is probably the drug of choice; either alone, combined with metronidazole, or as co-amoxiclav (amoxycillin and clavulanic acid). Evidence for the routine use of antibiotics and the actual regime to be followed is limited. Regimes vary from 24 h of intravenous cover to a more conventional longer oral course but, if healing is proceeding well, antibiotics can usually be discontinued approximately 2–5 days after reduction and immobilization of the fracture.

Avoidance of nose blowing

This is advised in patients who have sustained fractures through any of the sinuses or anterior cranial fossa, which applies to most midface fractures. The concern is that any forceful Valsava manoeuvre will force air and bacterial containing mucus through the fractures and into the soft tissues or intracranially. Theoretically this could increase the risk of infection, tension pneumocephalus or retrobulbar emphysema with proptosis.

With all midface fractures it is generally acceptable to permit unilateral gentle blowing of the nose without occluding the nostril being cleared. If the patient has to sneeze they should try to do so with the mouth open, a far from easy procedure for such a reflex reaction! Although these precautions are all designed to avoid a rapid build-up of pressure within the nasal cavity the actual degree of clinical risk is unknown due a lack of reported evidence. It also has to be accepted that this is a counsel of perfection in most cases. The desire to clear the nasal passages is very strong and it is very difficult for any patient with mid-face injuries to comply with this regime for longer than a few days, although this is almost certainly sufficient.

Oral and nasal hygiene

Effective oral hygiene plays an important part in the prevention of infection of a fracture involving the oral cavity. The conscious patient should be prescribed a 0.2% chlorhexidine gluconate mouthwash 3–4 times daily in order to reduce bacterial counts and improve plaque control. A soft toothbrush can be used carefully after meals, obviously avoiding any intraoral wounds. Patients whose fractures are immobilized by any of the methods used for intermaxillary fixation can also keep the apparatus clean by using a toothbrush in the usual manner.

If, for any reason, the patient is unable to cooperate in these simple measures the mouth must be regularly cleaned by the nursing staff, using chlorhexidine irrigation or sponge swabbing supplemented by tooth brushing.

In spite of the theoretical advantages of elastic loops when intermaxillary fixation is used, there is no doubt that wire loops are more hygienic and for this reason many operators still prefer them. The lips should at all times be kept lubricated with petroleum jelly to prevent them becoming dry and sticking together. If the lips are in any way excoriated or sore 1% hydrocortisone ointment can be applied with benefit.

Immediately following operation, saliva tends to become thick and difficult to control. This condition may persist for the first few days after injury. It is much more difficult for a patient to cope with this if intermaxillary fixation has been applied. The thickened saliva and congealed blood tend to block the interstices between the teeth and hinder oral respiration. The lips tend to stick together, which adds to the problem. It is during this period that good nursing can do much to aid comfort and rapid recovery. The lips and mouth should be cleaned with moist saline or chlorhexidine swabs at regular intervals and the lips regularly lubricated with steroid-containing ointment or petroleum jelly. Sodium bicarbonate solution is a traditional remedy for clearing away viscid mucous secretions.

Nasal hygiene is important with all fractures of the nose and nasoethmoidal region or when sinus drainage may be impeded. Regular saline douches help clear away dried blood and mucus, improve sinus drainage and hopefully reduce the likelihood of infection. Various proprietary solutions exist but a simple home-made remedy consists of one teaspoon of table salt, plus one teaspoon of baking soda to adjust the pH, dissolved in a cup of lukewarm tap water. This is gently aspirated or sprayed into the nasal cavity. Steam inhalations supplemented with decongestants such as menthol are also thought to be helpful.

Feeding

The problem of providing adequate nutrition following a maxillofacial injury depends on whether the subject is conscious and cooperative or uncooperative due to a depressed level of consciousness with or without cerebral irritation.

The conscious cooperative patient

The vast majority of patients with facial bone fractures are managed without the need for a prolonged period of intermaxillary fixation. This simplifies their feeding requirements considerably as they are merely required to eat softer foods than normal and should have no difficulty in maintaining their normal bodily needs.

Even when the jaws are immobilized by intermaxillary wires, patients can readily feed by mouth with a semi-solid or a liquid diet. An intake of 2000–2500 calories is adequate for most patients' nutritional requirements. However, a liquid or semi-solid diet is uninteresting and tedious to consume and for this reason patients should be encouraged to eat small amounts often. The balance of the diet should be decided in consultation with a dietician who will generally encourage patients to eat as much of their normal food as can be prepared by an electric food mixer or liquidizer. Milk and milk products are encouraged for regular daily consumption. However, these must be followed by meticulous oral hygiene. The diet may need to be supplemented with vitamins, iron preparations and proprietary high-calorie protein preparations. Every effort should be made to maintain the patient's interest in the diet by the use of flavouring agents and the food should be presented in as attractive a manner as possible. While the jaws are immobilized, a feeding cup with a spout to which a suitable length of soft plastic tubing is attached, enables a patient to feed by passing the end of the tubing through a gap in the fixation or round the back of the lower teeth. Flexible drinking straws are also very helpful to enable a patient to drink.

The unconscious or uncooperative patient
Fluid balance and nutrition

A fluid balance chart should be kept for all patients suffering from maxillofacial injuries until such time as an adequate fluid intake is being voluntarily ingested. As a broad rule the normal daily intake of fluid is about 3000 ml and the output is made up of 1500 ml of insensible loss by evaporation from the skin, sweating, and so on, and 1500 ml of urine.

It should be remembered that all forms of trauma and all surgical operations provoke a complex metabolic disturbance that varies directly with the magnitude and duration of the trauma or operation. This consists essentially of a reduced ability to excrete water and salt with an increased metabolism and excretion of potassium and nitrogen. The impairment of water excretion lasts 24–36 hours and is characterized by low output of urine of high specific gravity. The impairment of secretion of sodium lasts 4–6 days and after 24 hours there is marked lowering of sodium and chlorine in the urine. There is an increased excretion of potassium that lasts 24–48 hours due to mobilization and excretion of intracellular potassium. The increased nitrogen excretion is due to the breakdown of tissue. These changes are a normal response to trauma and in most cases the disturbances are slight and do not require any action. Most patients with maxillofacial injuries will have been on a normal diet and fluid intake up to the time of injury and are therefore in normal electrolyte balance. Usually such patients can return to an adequate fluid intake by mouth as soon as the fracture is immobilized and such cases present no fluid balance problems. In conscious patients the fluid intake can be left to the desires of the patient, as normal kidneys have the functional flexibility to excrete excess salt or fluid from the body. This flexibility is only temporarily lost following trauma and operation. Intravenous fluids over-ride the natural control provided by the patient's thirst and therefore the amount administered has to be accurately assessed by the surgeon.

In a patient unable to swallow due to the severity of the injury, considerable dehydration can occur in 24–48 hours, especially in elderly patients. If the patient is capable of taking fluid by mouth it is unnecessary to employ any other route, but if for some reason the patient cannot swallow, enteral or parenteral fluid therapy must be instituted. Injured patients also need early and adequate nutrition and fluid requirements have to be supplemented by a sufficient calorie intake to promote healing.

Enteral fluid therapy
Nasogastric tube

If enteral fluid therapy is required it is usually achieved by passing fluid into the stomach via a nasogastric tube. Considerable advances have been made in this area and traditional thick-bore Ryle's tubes, which are uncomfortable to pass, are not indicated solely to provide enteral nutrition. All the patient's nutritional requirements can be administered via a soft ultra-thin

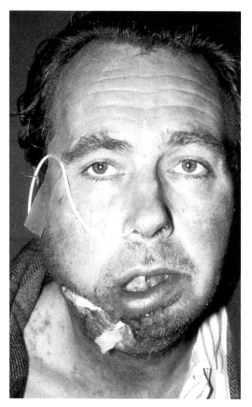

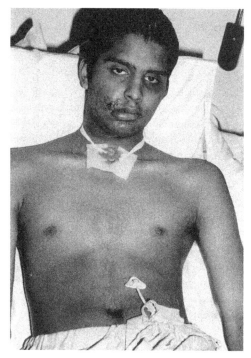

Figure 9.2 Patient with a direct penetrating injury of the oropharynx with a PEG in place to allow satisfactory feeding during the healing period.

Figure 9.1 Patient with a shotgun wound to the right face and mandible resulting in an oro-cutaneous fistula. A soft ultra-thin flexible nasogastric tube has been passed to permit enteral feeding.

flexible nasogastric tube using specially constituted food preparations pumped slowly under pressure (Fig. 9.1). If a nasogastric tube is passed in order to feed the patient it is essential to take a chest radiograph to ensure that it is in the stomach before any food is given. Occasionally these tubes are inadvertently passed into the trachea.

Percutaneous endoscopic gastrostomy (PEG) and radiologically inserted gastrostomy (RIG)

These techniques for the insertion of a feeding gastrostomy may be applicable in patients with severe maxillofacial injuries who require prolonged periods of supplemental enteral feeding for adequate nutrition. PEG tube insertion involves passing a flexible fibreoptic gastroscope to inflate the stomach and locate a site for insertion of a thin trochar through the abdominal wall into the stomach. A guideline is passed through the trochar and grasped by the endoscopist who pulls

it back through the mouth. The gastrostomy tube is then anchored to the guideline, which is withdrawn to pull the tube back down into the stomach and out through the abdominal wall. The stomach is retained in contact with the inner surface of the abdominal wall by a soft flange at the end of the gastrostomy tube and a retaining flange externally (Fig. 9.2).

The alternative technique of introducing a RIG tube achieves the same end by passing the percutaneous trochar into the air distended stomach under ultrasound and radiological guidance. The gastrostomy tube is then inserted through the trochar.

These techniques are equally applicable in the management of patients with severe injuries that interfere with oral intake and swallowing as they are for any other postoperative patient who requires a long period of artificial feeding.

Parenteral fluid therapy

Parenteral fluid therapy is administered through a peripheral or central intravenous line. The greatest risk with this form of therapy is overloading the patient while normal kidney function is temporarily impaired as a result of the trauma and/or operation. It is exceptional for patients who have sustained maxillofacial injuries to require prolonged intravenous fluid in the postoperative period in the absence of some complication such as protracted unconsciousness and loss of normal gut function. After any necessary infusion of blood or other fluid needed for immediate resuscitation given immediately after the accident, all patients should revert to oral fluid intake and nutrition as soon as possible.

Late postoperative care

Testing of union and removal of fixation

Fractures of the middle and upper face unite rapidly and clinical testing for union is usually both unnecessary and impractical. Fixation plates rarely need to be removed. The chief reason for removal arises where the plate is prominent or visible beneath the skin or becomes exposed intra-orally. It should be remembered that there is a school of thought that believes all plates should be electively removed. The arguments are largely theoretical and are not so far justified by clinical experience in maxillofacial injuries. Plate removal can sometimes be fairly difficult and a selection of screwdrivers may be needed to cope with the variety of screw designs in common use. Occasionally a plate can be partially osseointegrated into the bone.

Fractures of the body and ramus of the mandible treated by osteosynthesis will not normally have intermaxillary fixation applied other than for a short period to stabilize the occlusion and minimize postoperative discomfort. Although plates produce clinically stable union more rapidly than traditional treatment by closed reduction, some care is needed in the management of the early stages. Patients should be kept on a soft diet for the first 2 weeks and carefully monitored in order that wound infection, should it occur, will be recognized at an early stage. Plates that become exposed or infected will require removal. Larger plates beneath the mucosa are more likely to become exposed and in the longer term to become infected. All plates are probably better regarded as permanent implants unless they cause trouble. In summary, removal is indicated only as a result of infection, exposure to the mouth, close proximity to the skin or interference with the subsequent design of a prosthesis.

When intermaxillary fixation has been employed as the sole means of immobilization, it is left until sufficient time has elapsed for stable clinical union to be expected. This is generally 3 weeks or more (see Chapter 5). It is then released to allow the fracture site to be tested by gentle manipulation. If the fracture is stable in normal function, intermaxillary fixation is discontinued and the fracture examined again 1 week later. Some slight movement across the fracture on manipulation is acceptable when intermaxillary wires or elastics are removed. The amount of acceptable mobility is a matter of clinical experience that is soon acquired.

Most techniques for establishing IMF allow the elastics or wires to be removed without disturbing the fixation to the teeth. This gives the clinician the option to immobilize the mandible for a further period with minimal inconvenience to the patient. The rarely used Gunning-type splints for edentulous fractures are an exception. It is then necessary to remove the whole splint before the fracture can be tested; yet another disadvantage of this largely obsolete technique.

When the fracture is satisfactorily united the fixation apparatus is removed in its entirety. Wire ligatures and eyelets should be unwound a few turns to loosen them and the wire cut in such a way that there are no residual obstructions to smooth withdrawal. Nevertheless the process is uncomfortable for the patient and local anaesthesia is often required.

Peralveolar and circumferential wires are rarely used in modern practice. They are removed by cutting one end close to the mucosa and pulling sharply and quickly on the opposite end of the wire. Local anaesthetic is not essential, but it is crucial to cut the wire cleanly to avoid the jagged end of wire causing pain as it is pulled through the tissues. The mouth should be cleaned with antiseptic such as 1% chlorhexidine gluconate solution before pulling out the wire to avoid introducing contamination into the tissues.

Extra-oral pins are removed using the insertion tool in reverse. The skin surrounding the pins should be well cleaned with an antiseptic before removing. After freeing from the bone the pins should continue to be 'unscrewed' through the soft tissues to avoid the discomfort of simply pulling them out. Local anaesthetic is not usually required.

The procedures described for removing all these older traditional methods of fixation are tedious for the operator and uncomfortable for the patient, and are a further reason why these techniques have become largely obsolete.

Adjustment of the occlusion

Minor post-treatment malocclusions are common, but are rarely a major concern since slight derangement of the occlusion will usually be overcome by allowing the patient to masticate normally in the early healing period. Usually there is sufficient elasticity in the recently healed fracture to allow the occlusion to correct itself. Nevertheless slight adjustment to the occlusion is sometimes required. Minor disturbance of the occlusion can be treated by careful selective grinding of the interfering cusps. Special problems arise when only a small number of teeth are present in either jaw. In this situation the patient tends to assume a bite of convenience. Such cases should be fitted with partial upper and lower dentures as soon as possible to stabilize the bite. Patients with fractures of the edentulous mandible can seldom wear their original lower dentures and new ones are required when the fracture is healed.

Mobilization of the temporomandibular joint

Patients seldom have any difficulty in moving their temporomandibular joints even after a protracted period of immobilization of the mandible, and usually no special treatment is required after removal of the fixation beyond encouraging normal movement. However, limitation of opening may be seen following the raising of a coronal flap for fracture management or neurosurgical intervention because of subsequent fibrosis of the temporalis muscle. The function of the temporomandibular joint may also be adversely affected in certain fractures of the condyle, particularly intracapsular fractures. Minor post-traumatic disorders of the temporomandibular joint are probably more common than realized and the overall mobility and closing force of the mandible may be significantly reduced, even by fractures other than those involving the condyle.

Physiotherapy and rehabilitation

A number of neuromuscular exercises may be useful following repair of facial injuries. The precise exercise required depends on the injuries sustained. Custom jaw exercisers are commercially available and may help restore full mouth opening.

Following orbital surgery, prolonged use of eye-patches should be avoided and extra-ocular muscle activity encouraged ('eye exercises'). A minor degree of temporary diplopia is common and occurs as a result of swelling and muscle oedema. This should quickly recover. Patients should be encouraged to look in the direction that gives them diplopia as this may help in recovery. If diplopia is significant or persists an ophthalmic/orthoptic opinion should be sought. A corrective prism lens may be required.

Soft tissue injuries result in scar tissue of varying degree and cosmetic deformity. Lymphoedema needs regular massage to encourage the adjacent lymphatic ducts to drain fluid from persistent swelling. This is particularly common in association with periorbital wounds. Scars need appropriate support and massage. The use of silicone sheets and gels are often advised to minimize excessive scar tissue formation. In some reports botulinum toxin has been shown to prevent scars stretching by weakening the underlying muscles.

Monitoring of nerve damage

If the inferior dental nerve is involved in a fracture of the mandible, or the infraorbital nerve in a fracture of the maxilla, the damage may take the form of a neuropraxia or neurotmesis and the period for recovery of sensation will relate to the nature and degree of damage to the nerve. Neuropraxia usually recovers in about 6 weeks, but neurotmesis may take 18 months or more and complete recovery may not occur. Surprisingly, in the lower lip some degree of sensation always seems to remain since the area of skin supplied by the inferior dental nerve has an accessory sensory supply from the mylohyoid nerve. The area of numbness will also diminish owing to the phenomenon of 'recruitment' from the peripheral nerve fibres. The lingual nerve is seldom damaged in civilian-type mandibular fractures but if the nerve is severed sensation in the anterior two thirds of the tongue is seldom re-established.

Early microneural repair of both the inferior dental nerve and lingual nerve can be carried out by experienced surgeons. The results are sufficiently encouraging to justify the procedure in selected cases.

Care of teeth and supporting tissues

Fixation methods that involve attachments to the teeth need to distribute the load evenly to avoid excessive traction on individual segments of the dentition. Otherwise significant damage to the periodontal ligament will occur that may be irreversible. After removal of eyelet wires or arch bars vigorous attention to oral hygiene is essential and the patient should be instructed accordingly. Where teeth have been retained in the line of fracture, localized periodontal breakdown may need specific periodontal treatment to obviate further deterioration. Fortunately the periodontal ligament undergoes rapid repair after trauma and is reconstituted within a period of 2 weeks in the majority of cases.

Teeth, whether directly or indirectly involved in the fracture, may have been devitalized. Studies have shown that up to 50% of involved teeth undergo pulp necrosis. In the lower jaw such teeth are often in a sensory denervated section of the mandible and standard vitality tests are unreliable. Careful postoperative monitoring of the dentition is most important and unfortunately often neglected. When teeth have been lost, replacement by fixed or removable prostheses should be part of the overall treatment plan.

Further reading

Adeyemo MF, Ogunlewe MO, Ladeinde AL. Is healing outcome of 2 weeks intermaxillary fixation different from that of 4 to 6 weeks intermaxillary fixation in the treatment of mandibular fractures? *J Oral Maxillofac Surg.* 2012;70:1896–1902.

Bayat A, McGrouther DA. Clinical management of skin scarring. *Skinmed.* 2005;4:165–173.

Gassner HG, Sherris DA. Chemoimmobilization: improving predictability in the treatment of facial scars. *Plast Reconstr Surg.* 2003;112:1464–1466.

Jorgenson DS, Mayer MH, Ellenbogen RG, Centeno JA, Johnson FB, Mullick FG, Manson PN. Detection of titanium in human tissues after craniofacial surgery. *Plast Reconstr Surg.* 1997;99:976–979.

Reish RG, Eriksson E. Scars: a review of emerging and currently available therapies. *Plast Reconstr Surg.* 2008;122:1068–1078.

Rosenberg A, Grätz KW, Sailer HF: Should titanium miniplates be removed after bone healing is complete? *Int J Oral Maxillofac Surg.* 1993;22:185–188.

Wilson AM. Use of botulinum toxin type A to prevent widening of facial scars. *Plast Reconstr Surg.* 2006;117:1758–1766.

CHAPTER 10

Complications

Serious complications following repair of facial injuries are rare providing the fracture or soft tissue wound has been competently treated. Minor complications are, however, probably more common than is generally realized. Complications may be considered under three main headings:

1 Delayed treatment.
2 Complications arising during or soon after primary treatment.
3 Late complications.

Delayed treatment

Dentoalveolar fractures

Traumatized teeth may have been subluxed or otherwise devitalized. The crown, root or both may be fractured and with the passage of time this frequently leads to the development of apical infection.

Untreated alveolar fractures either unite in an incorrect position or become infected often with sequestration of detached fragments of bone.

Tooth fragments or foreign bodies embedded in the lip usually heal over and remain as hard lumps that may cause the patient some irritation. Although they are frequently well demonstrated on radiographs, they are not as easy to remove as they may appear to be for the inexperienced operator. Large or infected fragments need to be removed and are fortunately, in these circumstances, much easier to find through an intraoral incision.

Mandibular fractures

Whenever bone to bone contact is maintained at a fracture site union is likely to occur unless prevented by intercurrent infection (Fig. 10.1). When treatment of such a fracture has been delayed for two or three weeks it is still relatively easy to mobilize the bone at the fracture site and apply direct fixation. However,

precise anatomical reduction is much harder to achieve and bleeding may complicate surgery. Teeth in the fracture line at this stage are best removed, even in the absence of obvious infection. An infected fracture site will usually heal more readily after late manipulation if a drain is inserted for a few days. Clinically united fractures seen a month or more after injury should be treated as an established malunion.

Zygomatic complex fractures

If several weeks are allowed to elapse before reducing a fractured zygoma, the reduced fracture will probably be unstable because the fractured ends will no longer interdigitate well. This is due to osteoclastic activity rounding off the bony spicules. Some form of direct fixation will therefore be required. After about a month, it will be found almost impossible to elevate a fractured zygomatic bone in the conventional manner. However, the resistance to elevation is largely the result of early scar tissue formation. Surgical exposure at each fracture site and extensive sub-periosteal dissection will allow adequate mobilization and reduction even up to 6–8 weeks after injury.

It is well worth making the attempt at this stage, because the zygomatic complex will still retain its basic anatomical form. It is much easier, in these circumstances, to effect a satisfactory reduction than it is to carry out a formal osteotomy after full bony malunion with associated remodelling has taken place.

Nasal complex fractures

To obtain a satisfactory functional and aesthetically pleasing result it is essential that nasal fractures are treated soon after the injury. In contrast to the zygomatic complex, there is little advantage in attempting to treat a neglected nasal complex fracture after the first three weeks following injury. A better result will

Fractures of the Facial Skeleton, Second Edition. Michael Perry, Andrew Brown and Peter Banks.
© 2015 John Wiley & Sons, Ltd. Published 2015 by John Wiley & Sons, Ltd.

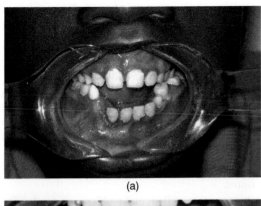

(a)

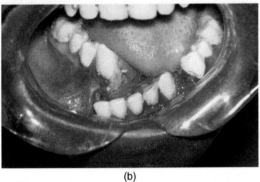

(b)

Figure 10.1   Malunited fractures due to late presentation. (a) Child with right parasymphyseal fracture. Union is rapid in this age group but refracture is usually straightforward. (b) Bilateral anterior fractures in an adult. In this situation, precise anatomical reduction by ORIF may be complicated by partial bone healing and remodelling. Arch bars and IMF may be needed instead or in addition.

usually be obtained by formal rhinoplasty at a later date. The exception to this is in more extensive fractures resulting in traumatic telecanthus. Whereas a late septorhinoplasty can be successful in restoring the nasal profile and re-establishing the nasal airway, it is less effective for correcting established telecanthus. The earlier a canthopexy can be performed the better will be the eventual result.

Le Fort I, II and III type fractures

When the treatment has not been unduly delayed, it is usually possible to mobilize the fracture, but this may involve fairly extensive periosteal stripping from both intra- and extra-oral approaches. It is usually easier to reduce the tooth-bearing portion of the fracture than the nasoethmoidal region. In some late presenting Le Fort I and II type fractures, strong and sustained traction by intermaxillary elastics has been recommended. Historically, even extra-oral traction was used in some cases. Newer techniques for callus distraction, using intra- or extra-oral appliances may have a place in treatment but require further evaluation. If the patient is fit enough for a general anaesthetic, operative reduction is always to be preferred and is usually successful within the first three weeks after injury.

If malunion of the fragments has occurred, a formal osteotomy can usually be designed at the Le Fort I or II level that will correct the occlusion. Such osteotomies are always more difficult in post-traumatic deformity than they are for the treatment of developmental jaw disproportion. Operative bleeding can be troublesome and considerable experience is necessary before embarking on such corrective procedures.

In cases where lack of treatment has resulted in a minor degree of 'gagging' of the bite in the molar area, occlusal grinding of the teeth or selective extraction and alveolectomy may occasionally enable an acceptable occlusion to be restored.

The treatment of severe facial fractures that have been allowed to unite in malposition presents a very difficult problem in reconstructive surgery and every effort should be made to effect reduction of such fractures before full bony union occurs.

Complications arising during or soon after primary treatment

General
Airway

Surgical treatment of a severe injury involving all of the bones of the face is a lengthy operative procedure and may impose further embarrassment to the airway due to swelling and the possible use of IMF. Close postoperative monitoring is important. If significant postoperative airway difficulties are anticipated a period of extended intubation and ventilation should be considered, or an elective tracheostomy performed before the patient is allowed to recover from the anaesthetic.

Bleeding

This can be significant depending on the extent of the repair carried out. Patients may have already lost a significant amount of blood at the time of injury and further severe haemorrhage during early repair may be detrimental. Fractures involving the nasal mucosa seem particularly prone to bleeding.

Cerebral

All patients with fractures of the face have sustained some degree of transmitted violence to the brain. Standard head injury charts are available in all hospitals to enable early detection of rising intracranial pressure and other signs of intracranial trauma. They should be used in all cases where there has been a definite or suspected period of loss of consciousness associated with the injury. When cerebrospinal rhinorrhoea has occurred, there is an added risk of infection that increases the longer the flow of CSF persists. Most CSF leaks after high midfacial fractures last 4–5 days and usually stop spontaneously. If a CSF leak persists for more than 10 days after reduction and immobilization, elective neurosurgical repair should be considered.

Displaced teeth and foreign bodies

Teeth or portions of dentures are occasionally inhaled and, when missing, must be accounted for. If this is not possible the chest and neck must be radiographed, and if a foreign body in the airway is present it must be recovered by bronchoscopy.

Fragments of teeth or glass are not infrequently buried in the soft tissues of the lip. They may be difficult to locate in swollen tissues but may become infected if left. If an abscess does occur, the site of pus formation locates the foreign body, which is then usually removed easily when the abscess is opened and drained.

Drug reactions

Allergic reactions occur from time to time, usually to antibiotics. These are fortunately in the main fairly mild but the clinician must recognize the complication at an early stage, discontinue all potential drugs and prescribe an antihistamine such as oral chlorpheniramine. True anaphylactic reactions are rare.

Dentoalveolar fractures
Pulpitis

Damaged teeth may develop pulpitis or apical infection in the weeks following fracture treatment. Such teeth are easy to treat endodontically in the absence of intermaxillary fixation, and relatively easy to treat after release of fixation if arch bars or eyelet wires have been employed. Any extraction should be delayed until

clinical union has occurred and even then carried out with care to prevent mobilizing the recently united fracture.

Gingival and periodontal complications

Some degree of local gingivitis is inevitable when fixation involves interdental wires or arch bars. This should also be borne in mind if acrylic resin is selected for the fixation of vacuum-formed plastic splints as a method of immobilizing a dento-alveolar injury. The gingivitis is usually not a serious problem and responds to local measures.

A more serious periodontal problem can result from applying too much interdental force to individual teeth from eyelet wires or arch bars. The lower incisors are most vulnerable and may be partially extruded or even lost. The complication can be avoided by spreading the load more widely and evenly by additional eyelets or arch bar ligatures and by avoiding the application of wires to suspect teeth. This potential complication is, of course, avoided by using direct plate osteosynthesis.

Mandible fractures

Mandibular fractures range from very simple to some of the most complex of the facial skeleton. There is a strong correlation between fracture severity and complication rate. The increased use of bone plates, particularly in the tooth-bearing portion of the mandible has, however, altered the spectrum of complications during primary treatment.

Misapplied fixation

Care is needed when applying plates and screws to avoid the inferior dental canal and to avoid damage to the roots of teeth. The risk of damage to structures within the body of the mandible is less when the screw engages only the outer cortex as is the case with non-compression plates.

Both rigid and semi-rigid osteosynthesis can distort the anatomical alignment of the mandible leading to significant alteration of the occlusion. Should this occur a decision must be made as to whether the malalignment can be corrected by elastic IMF and occlusal adjustment later, or whether a second corrective operation should be performed.

Transosseous wires are infrequently used in modern practice. Damage to internal structures should be avoidable but nevertheless ill-judged direction of drill holes

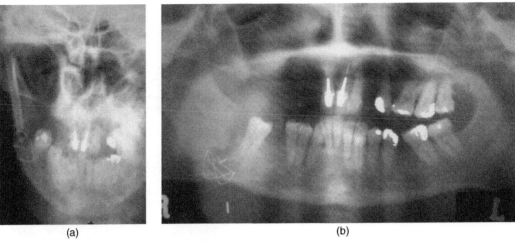

(a)   (b)

Figure 10.2 (a) PA radiograph and (b) OPT of an infected fracture of the right mandibular angle that has been inadequately stabilized by lower border wiring. The retained lower molar has also contributed to the increased risk of infection. A small sequestrum is visible on the PA view.

can cause problems. Similarly, circumferential wires are rarely used nowadays as they were in the past to fix oblique mandibular fractures or retain splints. If for any reason they are used they must be carefully located. A circumferential wire close to a fracture line may inadvertently be drawn up into the fracture giving rise to displacement of the bone fragments and damage to the inferior alveolar bundle.

The correct insertion of pins for external fixation is even more hazardous in unskilled hands. The pins often have to be inserted without direct exposure of the bone. They may impinge on nerves, blood vessels or teeth. They may split the bone fragment if inserted too near the lower border and they may fail to penetrate sufficient bone substance to remain secure during the required period of fixation.

Infection

Fortunately infection of the fracture site resulting in necrosis or osteomyelitis of the mandible is rare. Inadequate stabilization of a fracture increases the risk of both infection and non-union (Fig. 10.2). Mucosal wound dehiscence following open reduction and plate insertion still happens relatively frequently. This predisposes to localized soft tissue infection, particularly in the presence of poor oral hygiene and lack of patient compliance. This is significantly more likely in fractures at the angle of the mandible with involved teeth. When teeth are retained in the fracture line

there is always some risk of infection and for this reason prophylactic antibiotics should be prescribed. Lowering of the patient's local or general resistance will predispose to infection. For example a malignant neoplasm that is invading bone will both weaken the mandible physically and reduce the local resistance to infection. In these circumstances a pathological fracture may occur. Debilitated patients, diabetics and patients on steroids or chemotherapy are more likely to develop infected fracture sites because of lowered general resistance. Self-imposed debilitation associated with heavy smoking or above average consumption of alcohol, is also associated with a higher rate of local infection.

With the more general use of rigid or semi-rigid fixation for treatment of mandibular body fractures, the risk of infection has had to be re-evaluated. There is little evidence that retention of healthy teeth in a fracture line constitutes an increased risk of infection, although there is a general consensus that retention of a third molar with chronic or particularly acute pericoronitis should be avoided. Controversy continues to surround the question of removal of functionless third molars involved in mandibular angle fractures that, as a group, seem to result in a higher rate of infection than other sites.

A few important facts emerge from the literature:
1 Infection is almost invariably associated with a tooth in the line of a mobile fracture.

2 The incidence of infection is significantly higher at the angle of the mandible in the presence of involved third molars.

3 The incidence of infection is not affected by pro-phylactic removal of involved teeth, but in practice, prophylactic removal is carried out for the more suspect teeth. There have been no randomized prospective studies.

It is unfortunately apparent that evidence concerning the incidence of infection of mandibular fracture sites is still inconclusive and further evaluation is needed, par-ticularly in relation to retention of third molars, elective removal of plates, and the influence or otherwise of an intra-oral surgical approach.

Nerve damage

Anaesthesia or paraesthesia of the lower lip as a result of injury to the inferior dental nerve is the most common complication of fracture of the body of the mandible. The recovery of sensation in the lower lip depends on the nature of the original damage to the nerve. While anaesthesia is present patients need to be warned of the danger of burning or biting the lower lip.

Facial nerve damage may complicate some fractures of the ramus and condyle, either as a result of a pene-trating injury severing branches of the nerve, or blunt trauma causing a neuropraxia. In the latter event recov-ery of the resultant nerve weakness usually takes place fairly rapidly (Fig. 10.3). If the facial nerve is severed, microsurgical techniques may be successful in restoring function but it is most important to perform the repair at the same time as the facial laceration is explored and sutured. It is much more difficult to restore continuity and function as a later secondary procedure.

Midface fractures
Nasal haemorrhage (epistaxis)

Occasional troublesome post-reduction bleeding from the nose can occur, which is usually managed by simple anterior nasal packing.

Ophthalmic complications

The rare complication of retrobulbar haemorrhage after reduction of a fractured zygomatic complex, has been described in the literature. More commonly, extensive orbital oedema may occur. Either way, both can result in a compartment syndrome of the orbit and, if untreated, loss of eyesight. The signs and symptoms

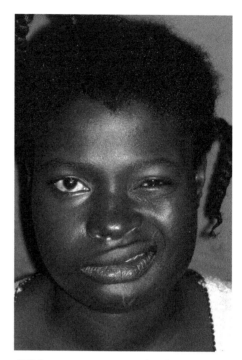

Figure 10.3 Lower motor neurone palsy of the right facial nerve in a patient who had sustained a fracture of the mandibular condyle. Conservative management resulted in complete recovery.

of this important complication are summarized in Table 10.1. The final common pathway has been sug-gested to be compression and spasm of the posterior ciliary vessels that supply blood to the head of the optic nerve, with the main blood supply to the rest of the optic nerve and retina being via the central artery and vein. Orbital compartment syndrome is therefore an acute emergency that may require decompression via a lateral or medial approach. Multiple techniques have been described and all surgeons who manage facial trauma should be conversant with at least one method.

Medical treatment should be commenced imme-diately while preparing the patient for surgery. This usually involves administering intravenous 20% man-nitol (1 gm/kg) and 500 mg acetazolamide to reduce intra-ocular pressure, and 3–4 mg/kg intravenous dex-amethasone to reduce oedema and vascular spasm. It goes without saying that urgent ophthalmic advice and assessment should also be sought.

The aim of surgical intervention is to decompress the orbit, and particularly the intraconal space. If an access

Table 10.1 Signs and symptoms of orbital compartment syndrome (retrobulbar haemorrhage).

1 Pain
2 Decreasing visual acuity
3 Diplopia with developing ophthalmoplegia
4 Proptosis
5 Tense globe
6 Sub-conjunctival oedema/chemosis
7 Dilated pupil
8 Loss of direct light reflex (Relative afferent pupillary defect)

incision has been used for initial treatment of the fracture this can be re-opened and blunt forceps inserted into the orbit between the inferior and lateral recti to enter the intraconal space. Alternatively the same area can be approached through a lateral canthotomy made with sharp scissors. A small soft drain should be inserted and no formal repair of the incision performed.

Blindness can also rarely occur following direct injury to the optic nerve. Deep extension of fractures to involve the orbital apex puts the nerve at risk during manipulation of the midface. This should be specifically looked for on the CT prior to treatment and patients consented for this small risk.

Abrasion of the cornea during surgery is inexcusable but can result from inadequate protection of a cornea, which has become unduly exposed as a result of periorbital oedema. Protective 'shells' should be inserted routinely at the beginning of an operation or a temporary tarsorrhaphy suture inserted. It cannot be emphasized too strongly that postoperative monitoring of the eyes must be carried out in all mid-facial fractures.

Inaccurate reduction

Inadequate mobilization of the midface fracture may leave it incompletely reduced. The occlusion and the accuracy of the midline must be critically assessed prior to extubation. In the anaesthetized patient intra-operative establishment of the occlusion may be inaccurate because of inadvertent distraction of the mandibular condyles. If reduction is incomplete and IMF is applied intra-operatively and then retained as part of the longer term treatment, the fractures may unite with the mandible distracted forward. When fixation is eventually released, an irreducible malocclusion will exist.

It is more likely that the mid-facial fractures will be immobilized by miniplates and the occlusal disharmony will only be evident after the intra-operative IMF has been released and the patient has recovered. Because the malocclusion may in part be due to muscle oedema it is advisable to reapply intermaxillary fixation and to wait a few days before making a decision to re-operate, as in this period the occlusion may come into line. Minor discrepancies can often be corrected by using IMF elastics.

Fractures of the zygomatic complex treated by simple closed elevation are inherently unstable. It is routine to inform the nursing staff of the risk of displacement of the reduced fragment should any inadvertent pressure be applied, and to mark the side of the fracture; although large 'hash sign' fracture symbols painted on the skin are to be deprecated, particularly when placed over the damaged bone itself. Patients have even been known to displace an underlying fracture while attempting to rub off the mark!

Nerve damage

Sensory loss over the skin of the midface is relatively common after facial bone fractures. This is predominantly due to neuropraxia of the infraorbital nerve and occasionally the zygomatico-temporal and zygomatico-frontal nerves. Surgical approaches to the midfacial skeleton need to be designed to avoid damage to the facial nerve particularly the frontal branches (see Chapter 7). Operative treatment can result in damage to both the sensory and motor supply to the forehead after a coronal approach. Upper eyelid incisions and exploration of the orbital roof may result in persistent ptosis that is extremely difficult to treat. Blindness and visual impairment have already been discussed.

Late complications

Complications from head injuries

Most patients with facial bone fractures associated with a period of loss of consciousness suffer to a greater or lesser extent from the post-concussional syndrome that consists of headache, dizziness, insomnia, diplopia, intolerance to noise, changes in disposition, intellectual impairment and intolerance to alcohol. Usually these distressing symptoms eventually resolve, but may become aggravated and protracted if litigation for compensation is impending.

An aerocele or a cerebral abscess may develop within a few weeks of the accident. Meningitis may occur as an early or a very late complication and occasionally epilepsy develops.

Complications arising from the fracture
Dentoalveolar
Devitalization of teeth
Useful teeth in the line of a fracture should be retained but there is a significant risk of loss of vitality particularly with mandibular fractures. Long-term follow up is therefore advised.

Loss or damage to teeth
Teeth are frequently lost or individually fractured after facial trauma. It is interesting that teeth are usually more highly valued by patients than they often appear to be by surgeons, particularly those without dental training. Adjunctive restorative dentistry is an essential component of the management of patients who sustain facial trauma.

Mandible
Malunion
Post reduction radiographs must always be taken and, should these reveal an unacceptable malposition of the fragments, this should be corrected as soon as possible by a further operation if necessary. After completion of treatment there should be no residual malocclusion. Inaccurate reduction of a dentate fractured mandible is always evident at an early stage when direct osteosynthesis has been used without IMF.

Postoperative use of IMF may mask an inadequately reduced fracture if the occlusion is not checked at an early stage after surgery because the mandibular condyles can be inadvertently distracted. Eventually when the IMF is released a degree of malunion remains. If IMF fixation is removed at the stage of clinical union when the callus is still soft, minor discrepancies in the occlusion will often correct themselves as the patient starts to use the mandible again. Selective occlusal grinding may help the process of readjustment.

Occasionally cases may be seen where inadequate reduction has resulted in gross derangement of the occlusion and deformity of the face. This situation may also arise when a patient has had no treatment at all for the fractured mandible, either because treatment was not sought at the time of injury, or because other more serious injuries prevented treatment or diagnosis. The mandible has an impressive capacity to heal itself and providing some bone contact is present malunion is more likely than non-union (Fig. 10.1). Gross occlusal derangement and facial deformity requires operative reconstruction usually in the form of refracture. Occasionally a formal planned osteotomy or ostectomy may be required. When the jaw is refractured at a late stage to correct malunion it is wise to pack autogenous cancellous bone, obtained from the iliac crest, around the newly approximated bone ends. If this is not done the diminished blood supply at the site of the original injury may predispose to further delayed union. Rigid fixation may also be required, possibly through an extra oral approach.

Malunion of edentulous fractures is the usual outcome of conservative treatment following closed reduction. Providing the malunion can be compensated for in the subsequent dentures, it is acceptable. Operative intervention and miniplate osteosynthesis of a malunited fracture in an elderly patient with a very thin mandible carries a risk of non-union without an onlay bone graft.

Delayed union
If the time taken for a mandibular fracture to unite is unduly protracted it is referred to as 'delayed union'. The term is difficult to define precisely as fractures heal at different rates but if union is delayed beyond the expected time for that particular fracture, taking the site and the patient's age into consideration, it must be assumed that the healing process has been disturbed. This may be the result of local factors such as infection, or general factors such as osteoporosis or nutritional deficiency. Providing the fracture site becomes stable so that jaw function can be resumed no active intervention is necessary in the short term. A fracture in which fibrous union has occurred will frequently progress to slow bony consolidation during the ensuing 12 months after injury. Fibrous union may be an acceptable result in an elderly edentulous patient. However, in a younger dentate individual, prosthetic replacement of missing teeth is impractical if any mobility at a fracture site remains and at some point non-union has to be acknowledged and treated.

Non-union
Non-union means that the fracture has not only failed to unite, but will not unite on its own. Radiographs show

rounding off and sclerosis of the bone ends, a condition referred to as eburnation. Non-union includes the condition of fibrous union referred to previously when there is a degree of stability.

Non-union may occur in a number of circumstances some of which are preventable. The theoretically preventable causes of non-union are as follows:

1 Infection of the fracture site.
2 Inadequate immobilization.
3 Unsatisfactory apposition of bone ends with interposition of soft tissue.

The remaining causes of non-union may be impossible or very difficult to overcome and are as follows:

1 The ultra-thin edentulous mandible in an elderly debilitated patient.
2 Loss of bone and soft tissue as a result of severe trauma, e.g. missile injury.
3 Inadequate blood supply to fracture site, e.g. after radiotherapy.
4 The presence of bone pathology, e.g. a malignant neoplasm.
5 General disease, e.g. osteoporosis, severe nutritional deficiency, disorders of calcium metabolism.

Treatment

A moderate delay in union is managed by prolonging the period of immobilization. Once non-union is accepted, and if the bone ends are still approximated, the fracture line should be explored surgically and any obvious impediment to healing such as a sequestrum or devitalized tooth removed. The bone ends are then freshened, the wound closed and the jaw is immobilized once again, possibly using rigid fixation. If there is any doubt concerning the health or apposition of the bone ends autogenous cancellous bone chips should be obtained from the iliac crest and packed around the fracture site.

If radiographs of a non-union show marked eburnation of the bone ends or excessive bone loss, a formal bone graft bone will definitely be required. It is important to eliminate active infection from the site before placing the graft, although if the obvious cause of the infection has confidently been eliminated, a bone graft inserted at the same operation will usually be successful.

Derangement of the temporomandibular joint

Conservative treatment of a fractured mandibular condyle frequently leaves some degree of malunion at the fracture site. Remodelling at the fracture site

Table 10.2 Possible complications involving the temporomandibular joint after fracture of the mandibular condyle.

1 Malocclusion.
2 Limitation of range of movement.
3 Displacement of the meniscus (reducible or irreducible).
4 Chronic pain associated with dysfunctional movement.
5 Chronic pain associated with osteoarthritis.
6 Fibrous or bony ankylosis.
7 Disturbance of further growth in children

is less efficient in the adult than in the child and post-traumatic temporomandibular joint problems are not uncommon. The main post-traumatic complications involving the temporomandibular joint are summarized in Table 10.2.

Late problems with internal fixation of the mandible

If possible, bone plates should not be placed near the oral mucosa as they will tend to become exposed. All bone plates may become infected some time after the fracture has healed. This commonly presents as an intraoral 'granuloma' over the insertion site. Removal of the offending plate will resolve the problem.

Transosseous wires are rarely used in current practice but those at the upper border may cause symptoms, particularly if covered by a denture. The wire is usually easily removed under local anaesthesia. Lower border wires sometimes give rise to pain and discomfort if the overlying skin is thin. In these circumstances they should be removed.

Sequestration of bone

Comminuted fractures of the mandible, particularly those caused by missile injuries, may be complicated by the formation of bone sequestra. A sequestrum may be a cause of delayed union but often the fracture consolidates satisfactorily and the sequestrum remains an actual or potential source of infection (Fig. 10.2a). In some cases a sequestrum may extrude spontaneously into the mouth with quite minimal symptoms, but otherwise a localized abscess forms and surgical removal of the dead bone becomes necessary. It is important to be sure that a sequestrum has separated completely from the healthy adjacent bone before surgical removal is

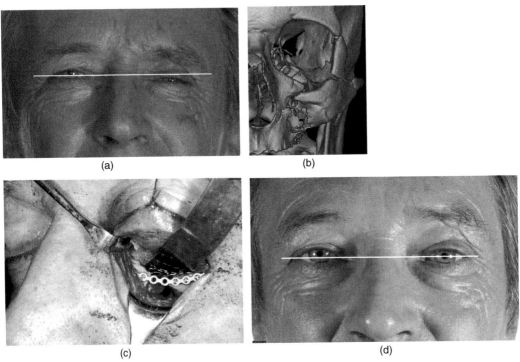

(a)   (b)

(c)   (d)

Figure 10.4 Late treatment of a malunited fracture of the left orbito-zygomatic complex. (a) Flattening of cheek with enophthalmos and inferior displacement of globe, resulting in restriction of movement and diplopia. (b) Three-dimensional CT image showing the malunited comminuted zygoma. Note rounding of bone at the fracture sites. (c) Surgical correction involved refracture and fixation, with titanium mesh remodelling of the orbital floor and medial wall. (d) Improvement in globe position and facial contour achieved.

contemplated. Very often an infection can be treated with antibiotics and the dead bone allowed to extrude spontaneously without surgical intervention.

Midface fractures
Delayed or non-union

Delayed or non-union of fractures of the midfacial skeleton is extremely rare but is not unknown. If a patient's central middle third fracture is treated by intermaxillary fixation alone, constant movement can delay union and in rare instances prevent it completely. Non-union may only be detectable when the patient applies the full force of the bite. Treatment is best effected by applying miniplates across the fracture site with or without a bone graft.

Malunion

If the fracture has been inadequately reduced, there may be bony deformity of the face. This may be entirely cosmetic resulting from change in the facial contour

or there may, in addition, be functional problems. The cosmetic and functional deformity may be more severe if there is associated soft tissue scarring or loss.

Zygomatic and orbital fractures

A depressed malunion of the zygomatic complex may leave the patient with a variable degree of cosmetic deformity. It may also result in disturbance of the movement or position of the eye causing diplopia. A depressed, healed fracture of the body or arch of the zygoma can interfere with the coronoid process of the mandible and restrict opening.

If such a depressed zygomatic bone is causing dystopia, diplopia or limitation of mandibular movements, a formal planned osteotomy will be necessary. Inevitably, because of remodelling of the contracted orbital floor, such an osteotomy will result in a considerable orbital floor bony defect. This will need to be filled with an autogenous graft or alloplastic implant (Fig. 10.4). If the depression is merely causing a cosmetic deformity, an onlayed implant of suitable alloplastic material may suffice. Occasionally if interference with mandibular movement is the main symptom, and the patient is not concerned about flattening of the cheek, a coronoidectomy on the affected side may be preferable to the more extensive surgery required to re-fracture and re-position the zygomatic bone.

Frequently in severe deformities there will be alteration of the orbital volume often with tethering and shortening of the ocular muscles. Expansion of orbital volume produces enophthalmos that is sometimes accompanied by diplopia. Diplopia or enophthalmos due to alteration of the orbital volume and scarring is difficult to treat. Bone, cartilage or alloplastic grafts placed within the orbit combined with ocular muscle surgery may be necessary to correct the defect. In this situation three-dimensional CT imaging and computer generated models of the skeletal deformity can be of great assistance in reconstruction; or even better the use of CT guided intra-operative navigation techniques.

Le Fort type fractures

Inadequately reduced fractures of Le Fort I, II and III types may leave the patient with an over-long face or flattening of the entire profile, the so-called 'dish-face' deformity (Fig. 10.5). There will be gagging of the molar teeth with an anterior open bite. The upper dentoalveolar arch may, in addition, be rotated to one side or the other and there may be post-traumatic defects in the palate.

Many of the inadequately treated fractures are those of the extended (craniofacial) variety in which the frontal bone and orbital roof are deformed. The initial severity of the head injury may have precluded effective reduction of the fracture. Apart from contour deficiencies of the forehead, the patient may present with considerable deformity of one or both orbits. Failure to correct nasoethmoidal complex fractures can result in a misshapen nose, telecanthus and obstruction of one or other nasal airway due to deviation of the nasal septum. Extensive damage to the cribriform plate or posterior wall of the frontal sinus can be the cause of cerebrospinal rhinorrhoea of delayed onset.

It can be readily seen from Table 10.3 that the reconstruction of the more severe post-traumatic facial deformities can present a major surgical problem. The principles of reconstruction, which may require a craniofacial approach, are summarized in Table 10.4.

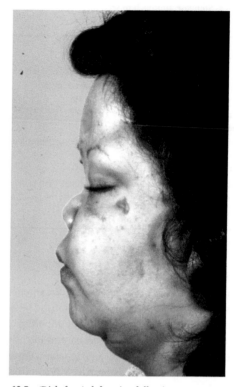

Figure 10.5 'Dish-face' deformity following an untreated Le Fort III type fracture with frontal bone involvement. The life-threatening severity of the patient's head and chest injuries resulted in an unfortunate delay in referral for maxillofacial management.

Table 10.3 Possible components of post-traumatic deformity in inadequately treated severe midface fractures.

1 Retrusion of upper dentition.
2 Anterior or lateral open bite.
3 Intraoral fistulae into nose or maxillary sinus.
4 Expansion or contraction of the orbital volume.
5 Orbital dystopia
6 Tethering of ocular muscles.
7 Depression of the nasal bridge.
8 Deviation of the nasal septum.
9 Telecanthus.
10 Obstruction of drainage of the paranasal sinuses, particularly maxillary and frontal.
11 Contour deficiency of the frontal bone with distortion of the orbital roof
12 Persistent cerebrospinal rhinorrhoea
13 Varying degrees of soft tissue scarring and mal-alignment

Table 10.4 Stepwise approach to secondary reconstruction of severe post-traumatic facial skeletal deformity.

1 Extensive facial or craniofacial exposure
2 Bony depressions corrected by onlay grafts rigidly fixed (Alloplastic materials are probably better than bone that can resorb)
3 Segmental osteotomies and bone repositioning
  a. Anatomically normal bone segments are repositioned following osteotomy.
  b. Abnormal bone may need to be replaced or supplemented by bone grafts
4 Rigid fixation to minimize late skeletal relapse
5 Soft tissue corrective procedures where indicated. (Soft tissue distortion is usually the limiting factor in restoring the pre-injury appearance.)

Ophthalmic complications

Residual ophthalmic problems arise from three main causes. There may, as mentioned previously, be deformity of the bony orbit with or without tethering of the orbital adnexae. This produces mechanical disturbance in the movement of the eye and in many instances double vision. Late enophthalmos is a not infrequent sequel of an uncorrected expansion of the orbital volume.

The function of the eye may be affected as a result of neurological damage. The oculomotor nerve is vulnerable during its long intracranial course and the abducent nerve may also be injured. If these nerves fail to recover completely the patient will suffer from strabismus, ptosis and diplopia. More rarely these nerves are damaged within the superior orbital fissure when a superior orbital fissure syndrome is produced (see Fig. 3.14, p. 35). If the optic nerve is also damaged, partial or complete blindness results: the orbital apex syndrome.

The third cause of residual eye problems stems from damage to the globe itself and its soft-tissue adnexae and may vary from disturbances in vision to diplopia caused by direct muscle damage. A small number of patients who have had direct trauma to the globe are left with impaired perception of moving objects due to delayed conduction along one optic nerve; the Pulfrich phenomenon. This can interfere with driving ability for example. Because of its importance, the phenomenon should be looked for specifically in all patients who have sustained midfacial injuries.

Paranasal sinuses

Severe midfacial fractures are frequently associated with comminution of the walls of the paranasal sinuses, particularly the frontal and maxillary. This may lead to obstruction of the ostium and disturbance of drainage. One or other of the frontal sinuses may then be converted to an infected mucocoele. In these circumstances functional endoscopic sinus surgery (FESS) is the best option to establish long term drainage. On rare occasions the sinus cavity may need to be obliterated or, very rarely, cranialized. In this situation it should be remembered that the pattern of drainage and loculation of the frontal sinuses can be confusing. One sinus may drain into the contralateral nasal cavity and total obliteration is needed to prevent further infection.

The maxillary sinus may become chronically infected as a result of obstruction of drainage, loss of specialized ciliated mucosa, or because of a residual oro-antral fistula. The sinus cannot be obliterated surgically so treatment has to be designed to eliminate infection and to re-establish drainage. Re-establishment of the natural function of the ostium by a FESS procedure is now preferred to artificial nasal antrostomy.

Lacrimal system

Partial or complete obstruction of the nasolacrimal duct may be a late complication of Le Fort II type and NOE fractures. The patient complains of epiphora and may develop an infected mucocoele, a condition termed 'dacryocystitis'. Referral to an ophthalmic surgeon is indicated. If the natural pathway for tears cannot be re-established by dilation of the duct a dacryocystorhinostomy operation is done as a planned procedure.

Loss of sensation

Apart from the nerves supplying the eye, there may be permanent damage to others. Anosmia is a distressing and not infrequent sequel to those fractures that involve the cribriform plate of the ethmoid. Anaesthesia or paraesthesia within the distribution of the maxillary division of the fifth cranial nerve is less serious. Sensation in the cheek, upper lip and maxillary teeth may often be diminished or lost.

Late problems with internal fixation of the midface

Plates or transosseous wires that have been used for reconstruction of the midface are generally nearer the surface than in the mandible and consequently more prominent. They may simply be uncomfortable for the patient, or become palpable or visible as projections. Those beneath the oral mucosa are more likely to become exposed and infected than those beneath the skin. In any of these circumstances the plates have to be removed. This is not always as easy as it sounds because titanium plates in particular have often become partially osseointegrated or overgrown with bone, requiring some patience and persistence to remove them. Plates on the frontal bone are usually inaccessible other than by re-opening a large coronal flap. An endoscopic approach to the area may be possible with the screws being removed through small stab incisions. The alternative is to make a larger direct overlying skin incision that rather negates the original cosmetically designed surgical approach.

Soft tissue complications

Scars

Many facial bone fractures have associated soft-tissue injuries and these wounds need to be carefully cleaned and sutured to minimize scarring. However, it has to be accepted that some individuals have a propensity to produce unsightly scars that are occasionally hypertrophic. Unsightly scars also result from contamination of the original wound with dirt, especially tar products. At first all scars tend to be red and feel hard to the touch but during the first year they soften and fade. Massage of the scar by the patient and the application of silicone gel are also helpful in this respect.

Hypertrophic scarring or keloid produces an ugly deformity but surgical revision may be disappointing. Repeated infiltration of the scar with triamcinolone 10 mg per ml can produce dramatic improvement in some cases. Whenever surgical revision is considered, it should not be contemplated until scar maturation is complete, which takes at least 12 months. It must be emphasized that adequate wound toilet and careful suturing of the original laceration can largely prevent unsightly scars.

Subcutaneous scarring can also occur in the absence of lacerations. It is important to remember that the energy of impact had to pass through all the soft tissues to reach the bones. These are also damaged and can scar even if the skin has remained intact: the higher the impact, the greater the potential to scar. Extensive surgical exposure of the facial skeleton and subperiosteal dissection may

also cause some late subcutaneous atrophy to a greater or lesser extent. These hidden soft tissue changes almost certainly contribute to the sometimes disappointing long term aesthetic results in severe maxillofacial injuries.

Limitation of opening

If there has been substantial haemorrhage within muscles a considerable amount of organizing haematoma and early scar tissue may be present in the postoperative period. Prolonged immobilization of the mandible with intermaxillary fixation will result in weakening of the muscles of mastication. All these factors combine to cause limitation of opening and a restricted mandibular excursion. In the majority of cases full movement is restored in time but as with other fractures, physiotherapy may accelerate the recovery period. Simple jaw exercises and mechanical exercisers may be employed with advantage. Very occasionally manipulation of the mandible under anaesthesia may assist the breakdown of scar tissue within muscles.

Myositis ossificans involving the main muscles of mastication is an exceedingly rare complication of facial bone fractures. It is believed that a haematoma occurs in the muscle, which organizes and eventually becomes ossified, a view that is supported by the finding of trabecular bone within the muscle mass at subsequent operation. Treatment consists of excision of the ectopic bone but the condition will often recur. The complication is extremely rare considering the frequency of mandibular injury and systemic factors probably play a part in the disorder.

Chronic facial pain

This is a recognized problem, especially after extensive injuries. The precise cause is unknown but it probably results from a combination of many of the previously mentioned factors. Patients are often surprised by the chronic nature of this problem but, by way of analogy, any extensively fractured limb will often give rise to similar long term discomfort. The face is no different in this respect. In many cases it may be more troublesome in cold temperatures and it probably reflects the under-appreciated soft tissue element of the original injury.

Further reading

Becelli R, Renzi G, Mannino G, Cerulli G, Iannetti G. Post-traumatic obstruction of lacrimal pathways: a retrospective analysis of 58 consecutive nasoorbitoethmoid fractures. *J Craniofac Surg.* 2004;15:29–33.

Herford AS, Ying T, Brown B. Outcomes of severely comminuted naso-orbito-ethmoid fractures. *J Oral Maxillofac Surg.* 2005;63:1266–1277.

Hosal BM, Beatty RL. Diplopia and enophthalmos after surgical repair of blowout fracture. *Orbit.* 2012;21:27–33.

Kloss FR, Stigler RG, Brandstätter A, Tuli T, Rasse M, Laimer K, et al. Complications related to midfacial fractures: operative versus non-surgical treatment. *Int J Oral Maxillofac Surg.* 2011;40:33–37.

Moreno JC, Fernández A, Ortiz JA, Montalvo JJ. Complication rates associated with different treatments for mandibular fractures. *J Oral Maxillofac Surg.* 2000;58:273–280.

Newman L. A clinical evaluation of the long-term outcome of patients treated for bilateral fracture of the mandibular condyles. *Br J Oral Maxillofac Surg.* 1998;36:176–179.

Stone IE, Dodson TB, Bays RA. Risk factors for infection following operative treatment of mandibular fractures: a multivariate analysis. *Plast Reconstr Surg.* 1993; 91:64–68

Index

Locators in *italic* refer to figures and tables (only shown where they fall outside listed page ranges)
Locators refer to adult patients unless otherwise stated

Fractures of the Facial Skeleton, Second Edition. Michael Perry, Andrew Brown and Peter Banks.
© 2015 John Wiley & Sons, Ltd. Published 2015 by John Wiley & Sons, Ltd.

Printed and bound by CPI Group (UK) Ltd, Croydon, CR0 4YY

27/10/2024

14580143-0004